ACHILLES TENDON

Edited by **Andrej Čretnik**

Achilles Tendon
Edited by Andrej Čretnik

Published by InTech
Janeza Trdine 9, 51000 Rijeka, Croatia

Publishing Process Manager Adriana Pecar

Technical Editor Teodora Smiljanic

Cover Designer InTech Design Team

Additional hard copies can be obtained from orders@intechopen.com

Achilles Tendon, Edited by Andrej Čretnik
p. cm.
ISBN 978-953-51-0264-9

For EU product safety concerns:
IN TECH d.o.o., Prolaz Marije Krucifikse Kozulić 3, 51000 Rijeka, Croatia,
info@intechopen.com or visit our website at intechopen.com.

Meet the editor

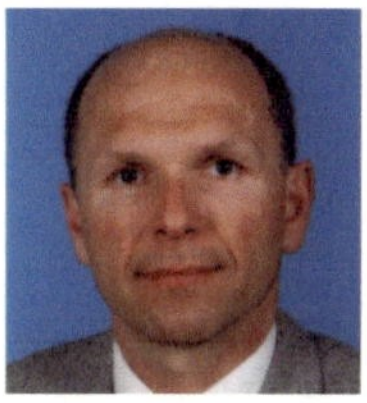

Prof Andrej Čretnik, MD, PhD, Med. Councillor, was born 1963 in Celje, Slovenia. He graduated from Medical Faculty, University in Ljubljana, Slovenia (1989). Dr. Čretnik became a Master of science (Msc) in 1999. (University in Ljubljana, Slovenia), Doctor of Sciences (PhD) (Medical sciences) in 2002. (University in Ljubljana, Slovenia). His additional education includes Royal Liverpool University Hospital (GB) (1994)(*Foot and Ankle Surgery, *Hip Surgery); Mayo Clinic, Rochester, Minnesota (USA) (1996) (*Spinal Surgery); Parkland Memorial Hospital, Dallas, Texas (USA) (1996) (*Pelvic Surgery), Trauma Shock Center, Baltimore, Maryland (USA) (1999)(*Orthopaedic Trauma Surgery). He is a faculty member at the University of Maribor, as well as a Senior Consultant Surgeon, Department of Traumatology, Surgical Clinic, University Clinical Centre Maribor, Slovenia. Dr. Čretnik is a member of Medicolegal expert (2004)(Ministry of justice, Slovenia), Medical councillor (2008)(Ministry of health, Slovenia), Medical Chamber Slovenia, Slovene Medical Association, Slovene Trauma Association (Vice-president), Slovene Medico-legal Experts Association, SQAA (Slovenia, National Evaluator), European Trauma Society, AO Trauma Society & AO Faculty (Arbeitsgruppe für Osteosynthesefragen, Davos, CH). He is also a chairman: Quality assurance committee (Medical Faculty, University in Maribor, Slovenia, Medico-legal experts committee).

Contents

Preface

Achilles tendon is beside a quadriceps one, the strongest tendon in human body. Its name arises from the ancient hero Achilles. His mother Thetis wanted to make him invulnerable by immersing him in the saint river Styx. As she had to hold him his heel remained unprotected and thus his weakest point. This was a cause of his death – he was hit in a heel by a poisoned Paris' arrow (led by a God Apollo) in the siege of Troy (term "Achilles heel" is so commonly used to describe the weakest point of someone). The name ***Achilles tendon*** comes from the story of the siege of Troy as well through the "barbarian" Achilles action when he attached the body of killed enemy Hector through "the strongest tendons in the body" to the chariot and drove him around the walls as a prove that he has beaten the greatest Troy's warrior.

Despite of the fact that Achilles tendon rupture is not a very common injury, it has always attracted a great attention. Hippocrates is believed to be the first who wrote about its treatment, but the first description of the Achilles tendon rupture can be found in the works of Ambrois Pare in 1575. "Modern" concepts of conservative as well as operative treatment with many proposed methods can be found since 1929 in works of Quenu and Stojanović. These works still attract attention and many publications still arise every year.

As very high forces are acting in this region (6000 N "in-vivo" and almost 10000 N "in-vitro" testings), a lot of "troubles" in patients could be expected in the Achilles tendon region. Differential diagnoses and current knowledge about this problems can be read in Section and Chapters of Achilles tendon disorders. The most commonly used term for different inflammative, degenerative and non-degenerative, reversible and non-reversible processes in this area is term ***tendinopathy*** nowadays. Clinical signs and symptoms are swelling, pain and functional impairment. Etiology is not completely known, unfortunately but many factors including genetic as well as extrinsic and intrinsic factors are already discovered and intensively studied. Effective treatment is on the way although unfortunately problems are not completely solved. New technologies with growth factors are promising but further studies with long term results are needed in order to confirm early findings.

Achilles tendon rupture could be entitled as the "final stage" of Achilles tendon disorders, although it occurs with no previous troubles or any signs in many patients.

Structure of Achilles tendon is already well known and various new imaging modalities enable us to visualize tendons and changes in them. This is beautifully described in the Section of Tendons and imaging. These could be of a great help in further investigation of the Achilles tendon disorders, particularly as the etiology of these problems remains incomprehensible. Crucial answer seems to hide in bindings (hydrogen and covalent) - what could be of a great importance in organization, structure and capacity of tendon to withstand burdening. Despite of a great knowledge and recognition of many important processes in human tendons, number, strength and maturity of bindings cannot be (yet) "measured or determined" and thus potentially problems cannot (yet) be predicted.

Once Achilles tendon rupture occurs, the most effective treatment is expected from the therapists. Despite of many different studies and meta-analyses, there is no universal agreement on the optimal management strategy of the acute total Achilles tendon rupture. Most authors prefer open surgical repair as it contributes to a low incidence of re-rupture, ranging from 1,4% to 2,8%. Strong repair with the restored length and optional augmentation offers the possibility of early functional treatment. As it is associated with significant number of complications (11,8% to 21,6%) as well as high costs, some authors advocate conservative treatment. High incidence of re-ruptures (12% to 17%), lengthened tendon and loss of strength are the main arguments for the opponents to criticize this method. Percutaneous repair seems to bridge the gap, combining the advantages of conservative and operative treatment, particularly if performed in an outpatient manner and under local anesthesia. As it has been criticized to be weaker than open repair with higher re-rupture rate, some new percutaneous techniques and one with biomechanically comparative strength and final functional results to open procedures are already in common use.

As the rupture most commonly occurs in "mid-aged" persons (in the most creative and productive part of life), the highest effort should be put in enabling patients to return to previous activities as soon as possible. There is universal agreement that functional treatment is the most effective way in this regardless of the used conservative or operative (open or percutaneous) method. There are more and more papers favoring functional conservative treatment, what (probably) yields to better results according to the lower re-rupture rate (but still higher in comparison to operative treatment) and better functional results. If percutaneous (or open) method is used as strong repair as possible (sensible) should be used as the repaired ends are better protected against gapping in functional postoperative treatment (what brings to better; final muscular strength.

Restoring the length and function (strength) is probably the toughest part of repairing neglected Achilles tendon ruptures. Despite of a very good and simple clinical (Simmonds-Thompson) test (no plantar movement of foot by squeezing sural muscles when kneeling over the edge of bench) Achilles tendon rupture could be overlooked in an up to 20% due to several reasons. In a final chapter of this book, we can read about successful restoration with the use of different other tendons or stripes. This brings our book to a good end.

Hopefully this short overview will inspire you enough to open and read our book.

Prof. Andrej Čretnik, MD, Ph.D., Medical Councillor
University of Maribor, Faculty of Medicine, Maribor
University Clinical Centre Maribor, Maribor
Slovenia

Part 1

Tendons and Imaging

1

Imaging Studies of the Mechanical and Architectural Characteristics of the Human Achilles Tendon in Normal, Unloaded and Rehabilitating Conditions

Shantanu Sinha[1] and Ryuta Kinugasa[2,3]
[1]*Department of Radiology, University of California, San Diego, California*
[2]*Department of Human Sciences, Kanagawa University, Kanagawa*
[3]*Organ/Whole Body-Scale Team, Computational Science Research Program, RIKEN, Saitama*
[1]*USA*
[2,3]*Japan*

1. Introduction

Tendons are known to have a profound impact on the overall function of the musculoskeletal system in their role as a structural link and force transmitter between muscle and bone. Their unique viscoelastic response under tension allows efficient use and recycling of stored energy during stretch involved in locomotion, modulating joint position control, and providing protection from muscle injuries through reduction of mechanical oscillation and shock. The study of the mechanical behavior of the Achilles Tendon, defined as the thick or external tendon running from the calcaneus insertion to the distal part of the soleus muscle, is of particular clinical importance, since it is known to be the most likely site of tendon rupture and tear in humans. This chapter will review the known mechanical, architectural and biochemical characteristics of this tissue, vital for the transmission for force generated by the muscle fibers to the bone.

1.1 Imaging studies

Real-time ultrasonography has become popular for in vivo measurement of human force-length relationships under uniaxial mechanical stress, an important parameter for the assessment of mechanical properties of biological tissues. Recent studies using this technique have shown that, similar to muscles, the mechanical properties of tendon tissue undergo substantial changes in response to both increased and decreased levels of physical loading and with aging and disuse and importantly, that the effects are partly mitigated by resistance training. Such changes in mechanical properties of tendons will significantly affect the overall musculoskeletal performance. However the exact causative mechanisms remain unclear. This chapter will explore the architectural and mechanical characteristics of the tendon that are likely to be modified as a result of chronic unloading and cause reduced force production of the limb and, how these changes can be reversed with physical rehabilitation.

Velocity encoded phase-contrast magnetic resonance imaging (VE-PC MRI) is another imaging technique used to noninvasively measure Achilles tendon strain and changes in its force-displacement relationship concomitant with chronic unloading and subsequent recuperation. This technique will be reviewed in terms of its ability to quantify the Achilles tendon Young's modulus (MPa) from a stress-strain curve. Higher spatial resolution, high tissue contrast and large field of view (FOV) afforded by MRI also allow one to clearly define and segment the two ends of the Achilles tendon; such capabilities are important for elimination of undesirable strain contributed by exogenous tissues and for consistent monitoring of the same anatomic landmarks over the duration of several months as required in longitudinal studies. We will review the results of several studies using the VE-PC MRI technique that provide evidence that tendinous tissues exhibit spatially non-uniform strain patterns and that this heterogeneity of the mechanical behavior of tendinous tissues is altered depending on the contraction type and loading condition.

1.2 Role of Achilles tendon in musculo-skeletal dynamics

A confounding feature of musculoskeletal system is the relationship between the calcaneus excursion (~30 mm) in the human ankle and the length of human soleus muscle fibers (~35 - 45 mm). In order to find the answer to the puzzle, theoretical approaches have been made to understand possible mechanisms which may explain how the human soleus muscle-tendon complex generates movements at the calcaneus that are almost equal to the length of its muscle fibers. Preliminary evidence suggests that some mechanical gain may arise at the ankle where the Achilles tendon is pulled towards the ankle center of rotation, creating an easily observed curvature in the human Achilles tendon. Curvature of the tendon even during relatively high-force contractions suggests that posterior movement of the Achilles tendon is constrained, even though there does not appear any definitive anatomical structure equivalent to the crural ligaments acting on the tendons of the dorsiflexors. Such a constraint would increase the proximo-distal excursion of the calcaneus relative to excursion of the Achilles tendon above the ankle. Elucidation of such mechanisms will be reviewed since these aspects influence tendon moment arm estimations and are critical when predicting mechanical behavior of muscle from joint performance or vice versa. With further understating of structure-function relationship, geometric muscle model will serve as heuristic purposes as well as accurate prediction of muscle function.

2. Mechanical and architectural properties of tendon and aponeurosis

2.1 Stress-strain characteristics of Achilles tendon

Muscle and tendinous structures (aponeurosis and tendon) make up a functional unit, the so called muscle-tendon complex. The in-series, morphological arrangement of tendinous structures within a muscle-tendon complex imposes a force-transmitting role on the structures and also take advantage of their elastic as well as the viscoelastic properties (Rigby et al. 1959; Scott & Loeb 1995; Zuurbier & Huijing 1992) supplementing the passive force transmission with energy storage and recycling. These mechanisms enhance joint performance and efficient power production (Alexander & Bennet-Clark 1977; Cavagna et al. 1964; Hof et al. 2002; Morgan et al. 1978). Therefore, the interaction between muscle and tendinous structures in a muscle-tendon complex has a direct impact on the performance and control of the involved joint(s). In addition, it has been suggested that tendinous structures within a muscle may possess active functions which includes resisting to stretch by producing contractile force, sensing mechanical load, generating mechanical signal and propagating the signal via the gap junction network which probably modulates collagen synthesis (McNeilly et al. 1996; Purslow 2002; Ralphs et al. 2002). The potential consequences for disruption of muscle function by changes in tendon seem almost unrecognized, perhaps in part due to our poor understanding of the structural integration between muscle and tendon and the degree to which their operation may be 'detuned' by changes in mechanical properties of either muscle or tendon. The medical consequences of operating outside of the normal boundaries of a well tuned musculo-tendinous system are also poorly understood, although clearly recognized in the persistent atrophy experienced in microgravity despite rigorous exercise programs.

Muscle force generation is length and velocity sensitive. The process is repetitive in the sense that muscles will always generate force based on their length-tension and force-velocity properties, causing tendon deformation. The magnitude of tendon deformation will depend on its own mechanical properties such as stress-strain relationship. Stress-strain curves are an extremely important graphical measure of a material's mechanical properties. Stress is defined by the ratio of tendon force to tendon cross-sectional area, and strain is defined by the amount of tendon deformation relative to its resting length.

Inspection of the shape of the stress-strain relationship in a soft tissue such as tendon provides insight into the unique properties of most soft tissues compared with traditional materials such as steel or wood. Typical engineering materials usually exhibit linear, elastic, homogeneous, and isotropic properties, which is reflected as a linear stress-strain curve for loads below the elastic limit. In contrast, biological materials often exhibit non-linear, inelastic, inhomogenous and anisotropic behavior. There are three distinct regions of stress-strain (Figure 1: stress-strain curve). The toe region typically lies below 3% strain, a region in which specimen elongation is accompanied by very low stress. This low initial stiffness of tendon in the toe region is thought to be caused, in part, by the straightening of the collagen crimp (Rigby et al. 1959) or shearing action between the collagen fibrils and the ground substance of the tendon (Hooley et al. 1980). The linear region is evident beyond approximately 2 to 3% tensile strain. The slope of this linear portion of the curve has been used to define the "Young's modulus" of the tendon. This region of linear strain extends to about 4 to 5% (Wainwright et al. 1982). The Young's modulus for rat tendon is approximately 1.0 GPa (Rigby et al. 1959). Permanent deformation occurs beyond the region of linear or reversible strain. The ultimate or failure strain of tendon is about 8 to 10% (Rigby et al. 1959). There is a considerable yield region in which tendon deformation is accompanied by very little increase in stress. However, although numerous measurements of tendon stress-strain properties were made historically (Woo et al. 1982), few were made under physiological conditions. This is because the in vivo tendon properties are more

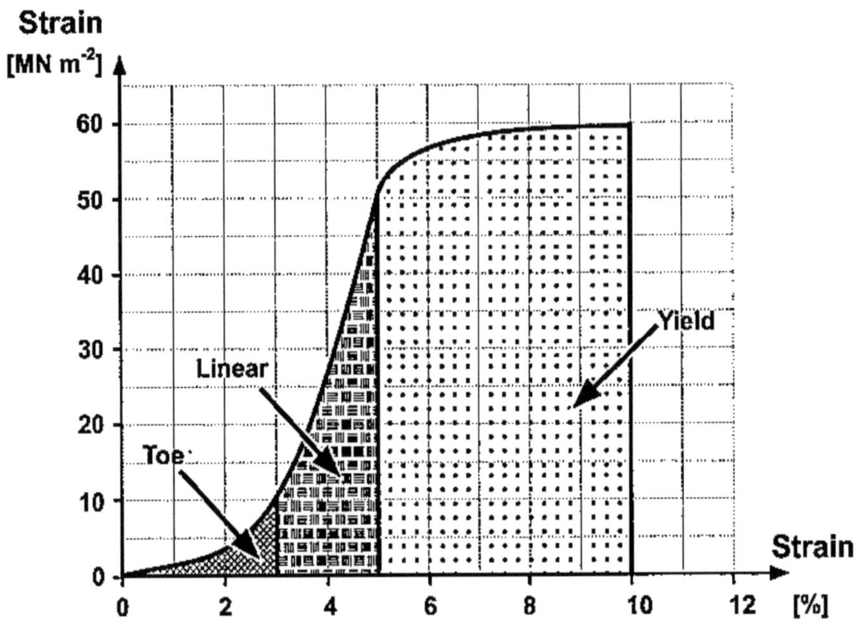

Fig. 1. Typical stress-strain curve for tendon (from Herzog et al. 2007).

difficult to estimate than the simple material properties of tendon tested in isolated condition. Several approaches have been used to define tendon in vivo properties. The examination of tendon properties under in vivo conditions necessitates the use of cadaver specimens. In one approach by Zajac (1989), estimates of tendon strain during muscle contraction were about 3% based on a literature values. Direct measurement of tendon strain during passive loading of a muscle-tendon unit (Lieber et al. 1991) and during muscle contraction (Leiber et al. 2000) yielded approximately similar results in that tendon strain about 3% at muscle maximum titanic tension.

2.2 Experimental determination of stress-strain properties of the Achilles tendon

Real time ultrasound has become popular for in vivo assessment of human tendon stress-strain relationship. The same general principles of in vivo tendon testing have often been applied with the aim of characterizing the mechanical behavior of the human tendon in different in-vivo situations and conditions. The results obtained vary greatly (Arampatzis et al. 2005; Bojsen-Møller et al. 2004; Kubo et al. 2002, 2004; Maganaris and Paul 2002; Muramatsu et al. 2001; Reeves et al. 2005). In young sedentary adults, for example, the tendon stiffness, Young's modulus and mechanical hysteresis values are ~ 17-760 Nm/mm, 0.3-1.4 GPa, and 11-19%, respectively (for a review see Maganaris et al. 2008). In addition, VE-PC MRI is potentially an alternative and supplementary in vivo technique. Tissue velocity measures of the tendinous tissues using VE-PC MRI enable us to estimate the Young's modulus during a submaximal contraction.

Using this VE-PC-MRI based approach, a new method was developed to characterize in-vivo and non-invasively, the mechanical (elastic) properties of the human Achilles tendon (Shin et al, 2008b). Achilles tendon force and calcaneus-movement-adjusted displacement were measured during a submaximal isometric plantarflexion in 4 healthy subjects, 4 repeated trials each. The measured force-length (F-L) relationship was least-squares fitted to a cubic polynomial. The curves were best fitted to a third-order polynomial, with non-linear "toe-region" at smaller forces followed by a linear elastic region. Typical error was calculated for tendon displacement at multiple force levels, stiffness from the "linear region", and transition point from the displacement point separating the linear and non-linear parts of the curve. Elastic constants of human Achilles tendon determined from these force-displacements curves, showed excellent correlation coefficient of each repeat set with the "average" curve, ranging from 0.89-0.99, 0.98-0.99, 0.97-0.99, and 0.88-0.99, respectively (Figure 2A). Qualitatively, individual differences were observed in the force-length profile in proportion to their level of physical activity (Figure 2B). The method yielded Force-Length relationships, stiffness and transition point values that showed good within and day-to-day repeatability. The technique compared well with the more conventional one using ultrasonography. Its reliability indicates potential for measuring tendon structural changes following an injury, disease, and altered loading. Both of these compliance related properties of the tendon have tremendous implications in the transmission of force arising from muscle.

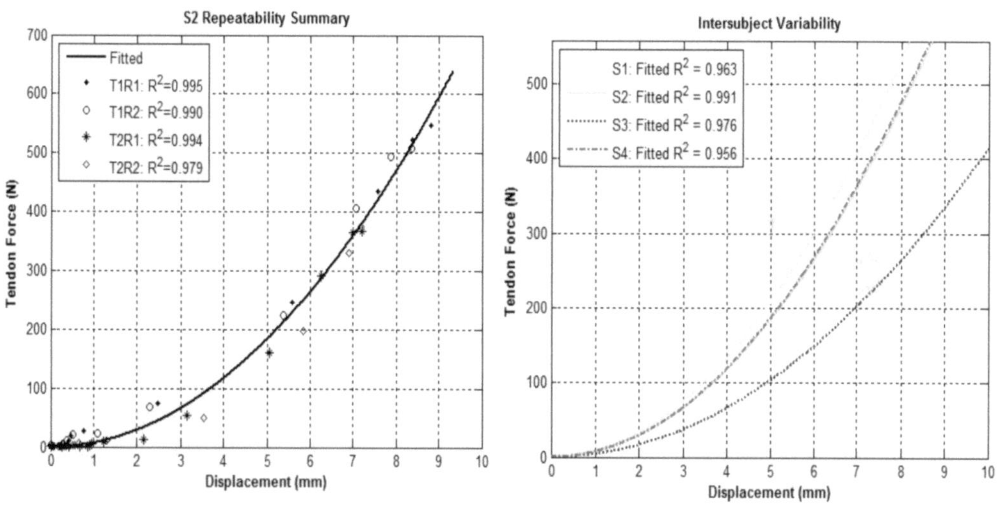

Fig. 2. Variability in Force-Displacement Curves for the Achilles Tendon using VE-PC MRI: (A) Interexam variability in one subject. Results from different trails are shown in different symbols. (B) Intersubject variability shown for 4 different subjects, with each subject show in different colors.

In a typical skeletal muscle-tendon unit, tendinous tissue commonly consists of an external free tendon, which is typically referred to as tendon, and an internal tendon, which is typically referred to as aponeurosis. The tendon connects the muscle proper to bone. The aponeurosis provides the attachment area for the muscle fascicles. In a recent attempt the separation of the mechanical behavior of the aponeurosis from that of the free tendon could be determined during ankle plantarflexion contraction using VE-PC MRI. One of the strengths of this technique compared with ultrasound technique is that it allows one to visualize the entire length of the aponeurosis, tendon, and even calcaneus. This allowed to the comparison of the stiffness between different tendinous tissues such as Achilles tendon and even regional differences along the aponeurosis. In a recent MRI study our group has also shown difference in stiffness between the Achilles tendon and distal aponeurosis of the medial gastrocnemius muscle (Kinugasa et al. 2010).

2.3 Correlation of structure of the Achilles tendon with its function

The primary role of tendon is to transmit the force of its associated muscle to bone. As such, the tendon needs to be relatively stiff and strong under tension. Herzog (2007) have stated that mechanical properties, such as fiber-bundle organization of the tendon allow for the maintenance of high tensile strength, with considerable flexibility in bending, in the same way that a wire rope maintains high tensile strength and flexibility as compared to an equal cross-section of solid steel (e.g., Alexander (1988a); Alexander (1988b) and Wainwright et al. (1982)). The significance of the observed tensile properties can be appreciated by considering the tendon function. Tendon must be sufficiently stiff and strong to transmit muscle force to bone. Ker et al. (1988) studied that relative size of muscle and tendon dimensions. The thin tendons require long muscle fiber, which allow for significant changes in length, to compensate for tendon deformation during muscle contraction (Ker et al. 1988). In contrast, the thick tendons deform less than thin tendons, and may not need extra-long fibers, indicating that the tendon dimension could have an impact on its mechanical properties.

Reconstruction of the lower limb muscle connective tissue from axial anatomical MR images (Iwanuma et al. 2011; Kinugasa et al. 2010) and from the Visible Human data (Hodgson et al. 2006) reveals a complex and somewhat consistent internal structure. The Achilles tendon is rather flat near its broad insertion to the calcaneus but becomes oval in the mid-region and then sheet-like as it courses proximally over the posterior surface of the soleus muscle (Figure 3, Hodgson et al. 2006; Kinugasa et al. 2010). The overall length of human tendon is approximately 68 mm and its width becomes larger as the region shifts more distally from the insertion of the soleus muscle (approximately 13 mm) to the calcaneus (approximately 28 mm) (Iwanuma et al. 2011). A small portion of the tendon and aponeurosis forms a ridge that protruds into the distal portion of the soleus and often reached the anterior surface of the soleus muscle. This structure is generally referred to as the median septum (Oxorn et al. 1998). The median septum extends toward the origin of the soleus for about 70% of the muscle length and is located in the anterior compartment of the muscle as this compartment becomes apparent in the proximal portion of the soleus (Hodgson et al. 2006). The posterior aponeurosis of the soleus muscle also remains very clear over the distal 60–70% of the soleus muscle and continues as a thinner epimyseal sheet in the proximal muscle.

A few studies have examined changes in tendon and aponeurosis dimensions under a human voluntary force exertion condition. In the transition from rest to maximal contraction, the length (superior-inferior direction) and width (medial-lateral direction) of the aponeurosis increases by 7% and 21%, respectively (Maganaris et al. 2001). However, the change in aponeurosis width is variable depending on the measurement regions. Figure 4 shows a 3-dimensional reconstructed image of the entire medial gastrocnemius and axial morphological MR images at 30%, 50%, and 90% locations along the proximal-distal direction under rest, at 20% maximal voluntary contraction (MVC), and at 40% MVC from

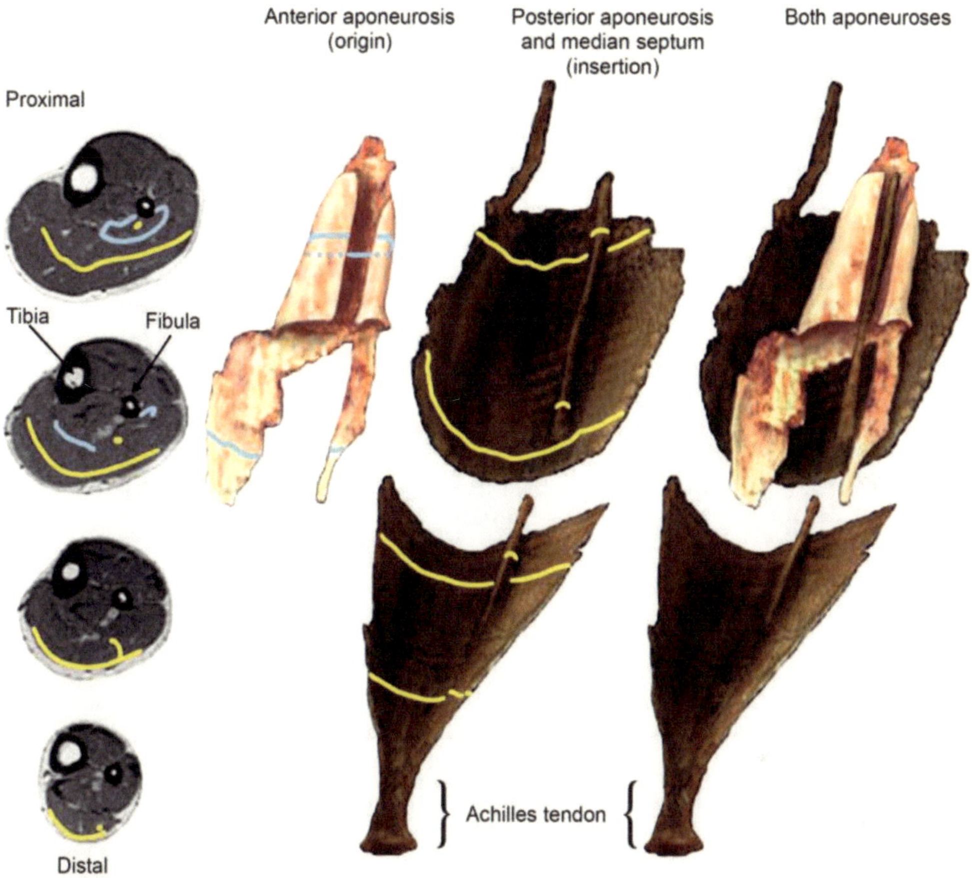

Fig. 3. Three-dimensional digital dissection of the soleus aponeurosis of origin and insertion from MRI images: These are views from the anterior. The gap in the middle of the aponeurosis of insertion indicates that the reconstruction was combined from proximal and distal images of the lower leg. The axial images on the left show the relative location of the origin (blue lines) and insertion (yellow lines). The colored lines in the 3D structures correspond to those in the axial images. A small band of the aponeurosis of insertion did not have a clear termination within the soleus but was contiguous with the gastrocnemius muscle (from Hodgson et al. 2006).

one subject (Kinugasa et al. 2008). At the 50% location, the deep aponeurosis exhibited greater sinuosity in the cross section as force levels increased, which resulted in a significantly greater segment length for 40% MVC (Kinugasa et al. 2008). In contrast, the cross-sectional segment length of the deep aponeurosis at the 90% location decreases significantly with increasing force levels. The contracted muscle is shorter with greater thicknesses in the proximal and middle regions. Presumably, the deep aponeurosis expanded in the medial-lateral axis. The distal region of the contracted muscle is thinner and the axial segment length of the aponeurosis decreases, accompanied by aponeurosis stretch along the proximal-distal axis.

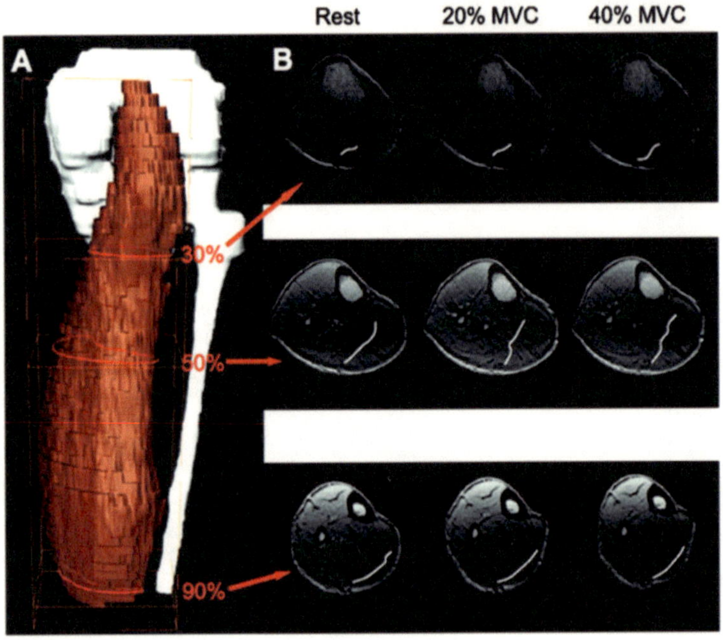

Fig. 4. Changes in cross-sectional segment shape and length of the deep aponeurosis. *A*: 3D reconstructed images of the MG, tibia, and fibula from a stack of axial MR images in 1 representative subject. Red lines correspond to positions at 30%, 50%, and 90% locations along the proximal-distal axis. *B*: axial morphological images at 30%, 50%, and 90% locations as indicated in the 3D image at rest, 20% MVC, and 40% MVC from 1 subject. The deep aponeurosis is indicated by white lines in these axial images and reveals changes in shape and cross-sectional segmental length after force production (from Kinugasa et al. 2008).

3. Adaptations of tendon and aponeurosis under unloading and rehabilitation conditions

3.1 Experimental determination of Achilles tendon compliance after unloading

Muscle atrophy is the process of loss of skeletal muscle tissue typically from disuse or unloading, which can arise from a variety of clinical condition including immobilization during use of cast, prolonged bed rest, and micro-gravity during space-flight. One intriguing characteristic of muscle atrophy is that the resultant decline in force per unit cross sectional area (CSA) is disproportionately larger than the accompanying decrease in muscle volume from atrophy. Our laboratory has reported, for example, muscle volume reduction of 6% accompanied by a force decline of 48% resulting from a 4 week unilateral limb suspension (Lee et al. 2006). Although reduced neural drive and a decrease in single fiber-specific tension are known to contribute to this phenomenon, recent evidence, obtained by MRI and ultrasound, suggests that changes in tendon mechanical properties as well as musculoskeletal architecture also play a role. Tendon and aponeuroses are passive elements of the musculoskeletal system whose main function is to transmit forces and displacement generated by muscle fibers to the bone. If the tendon stiffness is significantly altered, the mechanical consequence is that the passive elements will be required to undergo more strain in order to transmit the same force output compared to the pre-atrophy level.

Several studies have shown that unloading can have a significant negative effect on the mechanical properties of human tendon. Previously, the reduction in stiffness was reported mainly from ultrasound studies in humans (Kubo et al. 2002, 2004; Maganaris et al. 2006; Reeves et al. 2005) as well as in some animal studies (Ameida-Silveira et al. 2000; Woo et al. 1982). Recently, the tendon mechanical properties were measured with the stress-strain relationship established from the VE-PC MRI studies. For these VE-PC MRI studies, the Young's modulus showed a 17% reduction for the Achilles tendon (Figure 5, Shin et al. 2008a) and 29% reduction for the distal aponeurosis (Kinugasa et al. 2010) after 4-wk unloading. The extent of decline found in these studies is similar to that reported by Kubo et al. (2002, 2004), who studied humans subjected to 20 days of bed rest (-28%), but it is much more moderate than the percent decline reported in studies of 90 days simulated microgravity (-58%, Reeves et al. 2005) and paralysis (-59%, Maganaris et al. 2006). This suggests that the extent of stiffness decrease may have a direct correlation to the duration of unloading.

3.2 Physiological implications of changes in tendon compliance

A decrease in Achilles tendon stiffness results in a clear functional disadvantage. Decreased stiffness results in less efficient transfer of contractile force produced by the muscle to the bone, which leads to delayed motor behavior (Proske & Morgan 1987). Additionally, the compliant tendon results in a leftward shift of the force-length curve of the muscle fiber, resulting in a decline in force production for a given amount of fiber shortening (Shin et al. 2008a).

The exact causative mechanism for the reduction in tendon mechanical stiffness remains unclear. It is generally attributed to material deterioration, since the tendon CSA remains unchanged with chronic unloading in humans (de Boer et al. 2007; Kubo et al. 2004; Reeves et al. 2005; Shin et al. 2008a). However, this conclusion necessitates several major presumptions. The results of animal experiments characterizing the effect of chronic unloading on tendon dimension are inconsistent. For example, in animal models, tendon size has been shown to decrease (Schulze et al. 2002), as well as not to change (Almeida-Silveira et al. 2000; Heinemeier et al. 2009; Matsumoto et al. 2003), and even to increase (Kotani et al. 1998; Tsuchida et al. 1997) in response to chronic unloading. Interestingly, if the Achilles tendon of a rabbit is cut, glycosaminoglycan content and fibroblast number increase, and the number of small collagen fibers increase (Flint 1982).

Several human studies (de Boer et al. 2007; Kubo et al. 2004; Reeves et al. 2005; Shin et al. 2008a) have indicated that chronic unloading does not lead to significant change in tendon size, but dimensional measures were limited to a very restricted fraction of the length. Recently, in fact, human tendon size was shown to increase by 5% after 4-wk unloading based on relatively high-resolution data and sensitive procedure to test for significance (Figure 6, Kinugasa et al. 2010). One explanation may arise from further analysis showing that the entire length of the Achilles tendon and distal aponeurosis and median septum remained unchanged in cross-sectional segment lengths. This possibly indicates a slight increase in thickness rather than changes in the overall dimensions within a cross section.

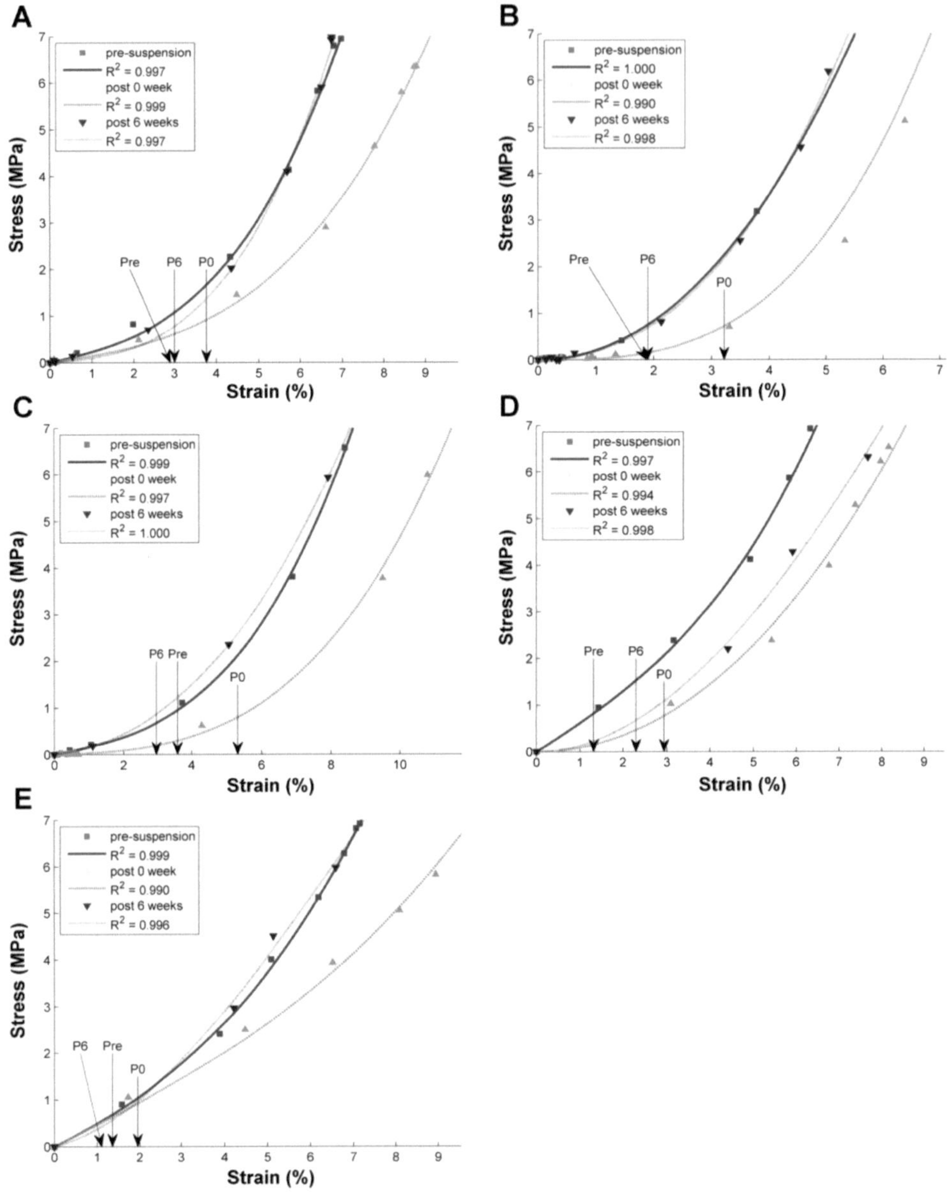

Fig. 5. Effect of Unloading on Stress-strain curve of the Achilles tendon: at pre-suspension (Pre), at post-suspension (P0), and after 6 wk of physical rehabilitation (P6) for five subjects (from Shin et al. 2008a).

This assumption is supported by some relevant findings including an increase in rat collagen fiber proportion (Binkley & Peat 1986) and CSA of ewe spinal ligament (Kotani et al. 1998) as a result of chronic unloading. However, animal data on the effects of chronic unloading on collagen fibril size, density, and number are conflicting. Human studies have demonstrated that, during 2 wk of unloading, there are either no changes or a downregulation of collagen I and III mRNA (Heinemeier et al. 2009) and collagen synthesis

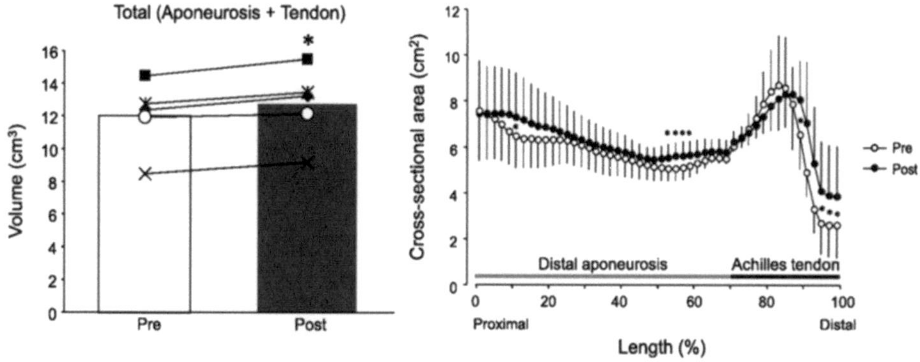

Fig. 6. Effect of 4-wk unilateral lower limb suspension: Changes in volume (left) and cross-sectional area (right) along the entire length of Achilles tendon and distal aponeurosis following 4-wk unilateral lower limb suspension (from Kinugasa et al. 2010).

(Christensen et al. 2008), indicating that the ultrastructure of collagen fibril might not alter with chronic unloading. An increase in the water content in extracellular space may therefore provide a possible explanation for tendon hypertrophy. It is possible that extracellular space could be increased in response to chronic unloading (Kotani et al. 1998, Tsuchida et al. 1997). Although the tendon hypertrophy observed may be expected to compensate for the reduction in the tendon stiffness, the absence of any significant correlation between the magnitude of tendon hypertrophy and reduced Young's modulus (Figure 7) seen in Kinugasa's study (2010) suggests that dimensional factors are not critical to the elastic properties. The literature seems to indicate that the altered tendon elastic modulus is largely due to material deterioration. Changes in the structure and packing of the collagen fibers (Danielsen & Andreassen 1988), such as loss of transverse bands of collagen fiber (Paavola et al. 2002), increased collagen fiber crimping (Patterson-Kane 1997), and reduction in the covalent intramolucular cross-links (Bailey 2001), may generally be considered to be factors in the alteration of tendon material properties.

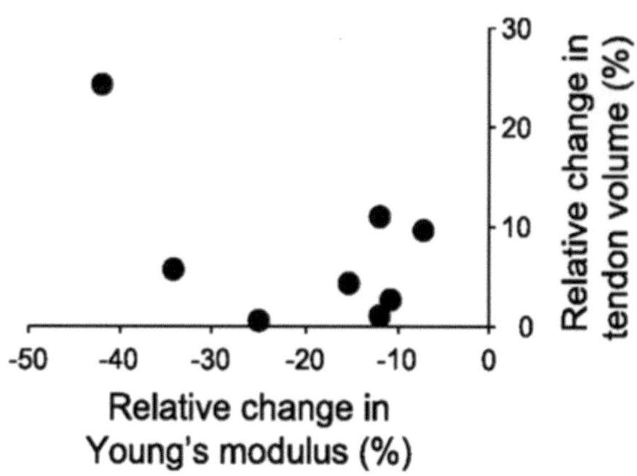

Fig. 7. Relationship between relative changes in volume and Young's modulus of Achilles tendon and distal aponeurosis after 4 wk of unilateral lower limb suspension. The regression line is not shown since the relationship was found to be insignificant (from Kinugasa et al. 2010).

The effects of unloading or disuse were demonstrated by reduction of the muscle force. The recovery of muscle volume and force with a chronic rehabilitation are well-documented in literature (Berg et al. 1991; Lee et al. 2006; Maclntyre et al. 2005), but to our knowledge, there is only one study which investigated changes in tendon mechanical properties with physical rehabilitation. Shin et al. (2008a) investigated the change in the Young's modulus in response to 6 wk of physical rehabilitation (six exercise; 1) warm-up, 2) strength, 3) balance, 4) stretching, 5) cool-down, 6) post-evaluation) after 4 wk of limb suspension. The Young's modulus was decreased by 17% following 4-wk unloading and returned to the pre-loading level at the end of 6-wk of physical rehabilitation (Figure 5).

4. Amplification of ankle rotation by deformation of Achilles tendon

4.1 Experimental determination of amplification factor

In-vivo measurements of muscle shortening during plantarflexion / dorsiflexion movements of the ankle show that the distance moved by the calcaneus exceeds the shortening of the muscle fibers (Hodgson et al. 2006). Thus, mechanisms must exist between the muscle fiber and calcaneus which amplify the muscle fiber length changes. One such system appears to be the internal mechanics of the muscle which prevents changes in aponeurosis separation as the muscle lengthens and shortens. We have hypothesized a second system operating at the ankle. The observed curvature of the Achilles tendon under load indicates the presence of a mechanical constraint close to the ankle which limits posterior movement of the tendon as the ankle rotates. Mechanical analysis of such a constraint suggests that it would modify the relationship between muscle shortening and ankle rotation, adding more amplification to the translation of muscle fiber shortening to ankle rotation (Hodgson et al. 2006). Although no structure is readily apparent, the observation of tendon curvature indicates that a force component perpendicular to the tendon load axis is present to displace the tendon from the linear orientation which it would

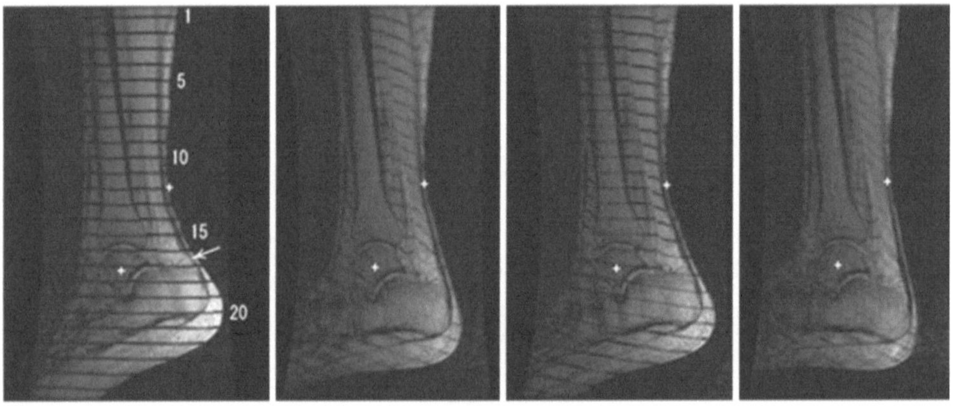

Fig. 8. Spin-tagged sagittal images showing the rotation of the foot during passive dorsiflexion of the foot (left to right): White crosses indicate the ankle center of rotation and the region above the ankle where posterior movement of the tendon appears to be prevented. The first panel identifies the tag-line numbers and the arrow indicates the point where the calcaneus meets the Achilles tendon. Movement of the Achilles tendon and aponeurosis was measured by noting its intersection with each tag line in several frames.

adopt with tensile loading alone. This prediction has been tested by comparing the displacement of the aponeuroses above the ankle and the movement at different points along the length of the Achillles tendon and calcaneous as the subject's foot was moved through ~30° by the motor at a cycle rate of 30° s^{-1}, with the subject exerting 40% MVC. On an oblique sagittal image of the lower leg in which the entire length of the aponeurosis and tendon could be visualized, the intersection of spin tag lines in the soleus muscle and the Achilles tendon / aponeurosis was detected, and these points of intersection were tracked in successive frames of the cine-MRI data (Figure 8). Additionally, the location of the apparent deviation of the Achilles tendon from a straight line was noted on each frame.

Several points on the foot were also tracked and used to determine the center of rotation of the ankle. In Fig. 9, which demonstrates the geometry of ankle rotations, Point X is the MG musculo-tendinous junction, Point Y → point where posterior movement of the Achilles tendon is prevented, Point Z → the junction between Achilles tendon and calcaneus, Point C → the ankle center of rotation; Line CZ → lever arm upon which the Achilles tendon acts, Line CB → the Achilles tendon moment arm which is different from CZ because the Achilles

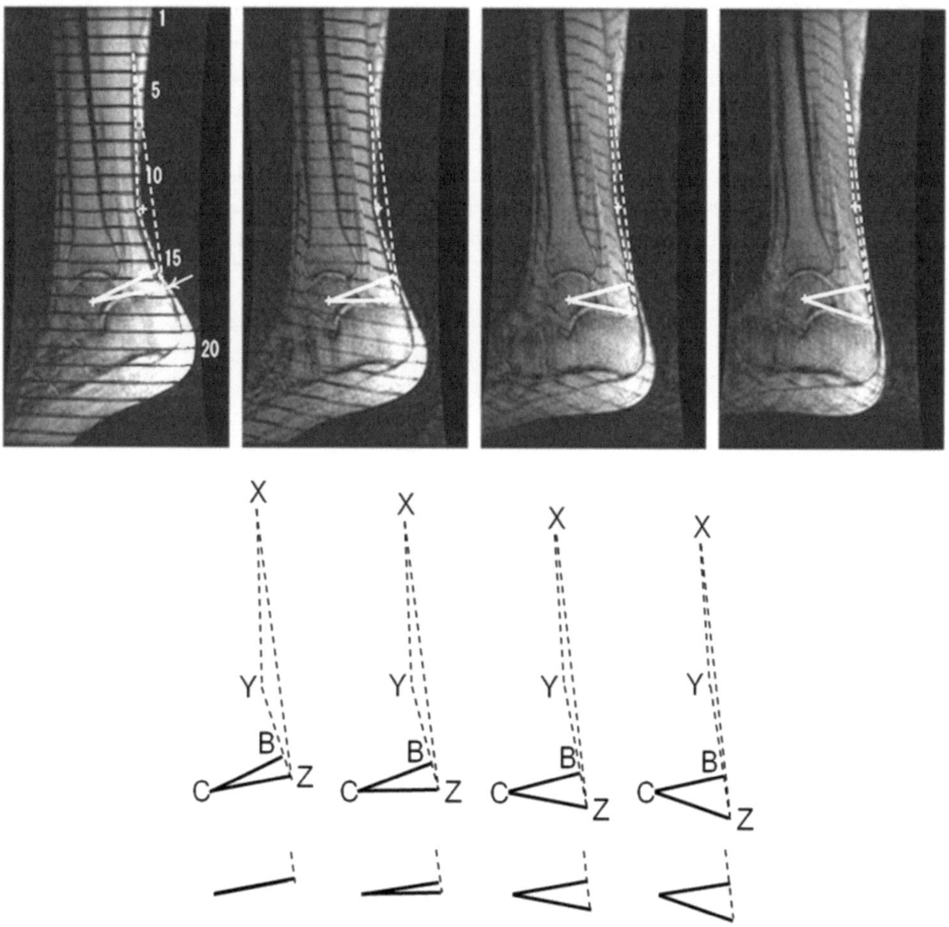

Fig. 9. Geometry of ankle rotation due to restriction of posterior movement of the Achilles tendon.

tendon pulls at an angle to CZ, Line XZ → the distance between the MG musculo-tendinous junction and calcaneus, Lines XY and YZ indicate the path of the Achilles tendon, Length XY+YZ represents the length of the Achilles tendon. The geometry of triangle XYZ implies that line XY lengthens as the ankle dorsiflexes (left to right in figure). Thus point Z moves a greater distance than point X, even if tendon length remains constant. Moment arm BC equates to lever arm length CZ multiplied by Cos angle BCZ. Angle BCZ increases with dorsiflexion, therefore the Achilles tendon moment arm must decrease with dorsiflexion. The lower row of diagrams on the right illustrates the greater change in moment arm which would occur without the Achilles tendon constraint.

4.2 Physiological implications of amplification factor

Figure 10 illustrates that the constraint to the posterior movement of the Achilles tendon reduces the tendon moment arm at the ankle over a wide range of ankle angles. A shorter moment arm increases the ankle rotation for a given change in muscle length. The range of moment arm change is also reduced significantly, possibly easing the challenge of controlling ankle torque at different ankle angles. The calculated lever arm length from the ankle center of rotation to the calcaneo-tendinous junction was 53.1 +/- 3.8 (SD, range 50.4 – 58.6) mm. The actual moment arm was always less than this value due to the anatomical relationship between the ankle and the Achilles tendon. Restriction of the outward movement of the Achilles tendon always resulted in an acute angle between the direction of tendon pull and the line between the ankle center of rotation and the calcaneo-tendinous junction. The moment arm is modified by the sine of this angle and is correctly measured by the minimum distance between a line through the Achilles tendon and the ankle center of rotation (Rugg et al. 1990).

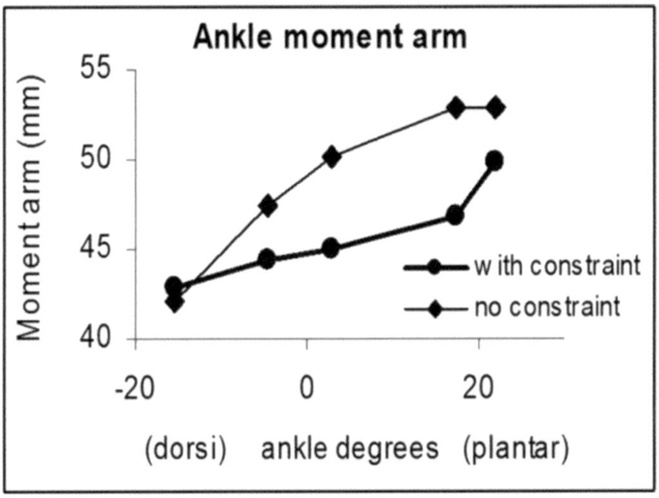

Fig. 10. Achilles tendon moment arm: The moment arm measured from MRI data (with constraint) is shown along with a theoretical moment arm based upon the Achilles tendon lever arm and a constant direction of pull set to the direction measured at full dorsiflexion (no constraint). The lack of constraint would also require the Achilles tendon to move posteriorly by ~1.5 cm.

Figure 11 demonstrates that the tags on the calcaneus have greater displacement relative to the tags on the aponeurosis, illustrating the amplification of tendon movement initially postulated. An unstrained posterior aponeurosis would result in all tag lines displacing by the same amount. Experimental observations confirmed previous observations that the aponeurosis does not move uniformly, exhibiting displacements which suggest some regions of the aponeurosis stretch while other regions undergo compression (Figure 10). Furthermore, some tags on the calcaneus showed a greater displacement than the displacement of the aponeurosis, consistent with the well recognized phenomenon that Achilles tendon stretches under load.

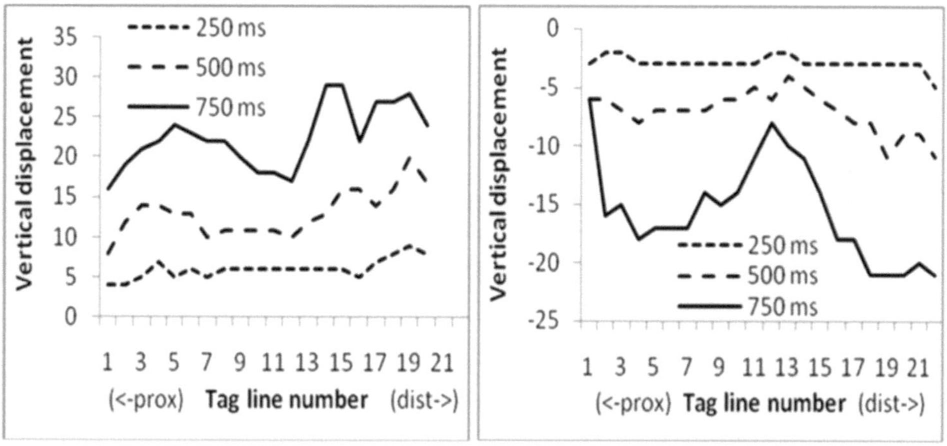

Fig. 11. Vertical displacement of tags at various stages of the plantarflexion (right column) / dorsiflexion cycle (left column). Note the greater displacement of tags on the calcaneus relative to tags on the aponeurosis, illustrating the amplification of tendon movement. Note also the uneven displacement along the aponeurosis, indicating regions of stretch and compression. The line style identifies the delay from the beginning of the movement and shows a progressive displacement of each ROI from the rest position (0). The most proximal region of the muscle is on the left of each graph and the calcaneus locations are on the right.

The alternative explanation for the differences between calcaneus and aponeurosis displacement may be an amplification mechanism due to the constraint on posterior movement of the Achilles tendon. These MRI experiments suggest that the major point of action of this constraint is 61.6 +/- 5.1 (SD, range 52.7 -65.6) mm superior to and 33.5 +/- 6.9 mm posterior to the ankle center of rotation.

The mechanism amplifies the influence of muscle shortening upon ankle rotation and decreases the Achilles tendon moment arm over much of the ankle range of movement. The data indicate that attempts to measure Achilles tendon length changes by measuring the distance between the musculo-tendinous junction and the calcaneus must also take into account the curvature of the tendon and any changes in curvature which arise from a change in ankle angle. Computations of the potential amplification by this configuration suggests a maximum gain of ~1.1 (Hodgson et al. 2006). While apparently quite small, this could have a significant impact on experimentally observed Achilles tendon strain. For example, ultrasound measurements of aponeurosis excursion during a maximum voluntary contraction typically report a displacement of 20 - 30 mm. If a significant proportion of this movement involves rotation of the ankle, this could account for a significant portion of the observed strain.

5. Conclusion

It is widely recognized that our muscular system changes its properties in response to altered mechanical loading. Previous studies have documented deleterious changes in muscle following chronic unloading, while recent studies provide information of significant changes in tendinous structures within the muscle. Recent work in our laboratory (Finni et al. 2003) in addition to work of others (Gans 1982) has demonstrated a significance of muscular structural organization. We believe the integrated structure of muscle and tendon is specifically tuned to the normal operating environment and normal physiological state. A better understanding of this interaction between muscle and tendon and their co-dependence in maintaining normal physiological function is essential, as is a better understanding of how unloading and atrophy disrupt normal function. One of the main objectives of our group's research has been to investigate the effects of chronic unloading on the mechanical properties of tendinous structures in in-vivo human skeletal muscles and furthermore, to gain insight into the possible mechanism(s) of undesirable adaptations of human muscular-tendinous structures occurring secondary to decrease in mechanical loading.

6. Acknowledgement

This study was supported in part by National Institute of Arthritis and Musculoskeletal and Skin Diseases Grant 2R01-AR-53343-05A1, USA.

7. References

Alexander, RM, Bennet-Clark HC. Storage of elastic strain energy in muscle and other tissues. *Nature* 265: 114–117, 1977.

Alexander RM. The spring in your step: the role of elastic mechanisms in human running. Biomechanics XI-A (eds. De Groot G, Hollander AP, Huijing PA, and van Ingen Schenau GJ). Free University Press, Amsterdam, 17–25, 1988a.

Alexander RM. Elastic Mechanisms in Animal Movement. Cambridge University Press, Cambridge, 1988b.

Arampatzis A, Stafilidis S, DeMonte G, Karamanidis K, Morey-Klapsing G, Brüggemann GP. Strain and elongation of the human gastrocnemius tendon and aponeurosis during maximal plantarflexion effort. *J Biomech* 38: 833–841, 2005.

Almeida-Silveira MI, Lambertz D, Perot C, Goubel F. Changes in stiffness induced by hindlimb suspension in rat Achilles tendon. *Eur J Appl Physiol* 81: 252–257, 2000.

Bailey AJ. Molecular mechanisms of ageing in connective tissues. *Mech Ageing Dev* 122: 735–755, 2001.

Berg HE, Dudley GA, Haggmark T, Ohlsen H, Tesch PA. Effects of lower limb unloading on skeletal muscle mass and function in humans. *J Appl Physiol* 70: 1882-1885, 1991.

Binkley JM, Peat M. The effects of immobilization on the ultrastructure and mechanical properties of the medial collateral ligament of rats. *Clin Orthop Relat Res* 203: 301-308, 1986.

Bojsen-Møller J, Hansen P, Aagaard P, Svantesson U, Kjaer M, Magnusson SP. Differential displacement of the human soleus and medial gastrocnemius aponeuroses during isometric plantar flexor contractions in vivo. *J Appl Physiol* 97: 1908-1914, 2004.

Cavagna GA, Saibene FP, Margaria R. Mechanical work in running. *J Appl Physiol* 19: 249-256, 1964.

Christensen B, Dyrberg E, Aagaard P, Kjaer M, Langberg H. Short-term immobilization and recovery affect skeletal muscle but not collagen tissue turnover in humans. *J Appl Physiol* 105: 1845-1851, 2008.

Danielsen CC, Andreassen TT. Mechanical properties of rat tail tendon in relation to proximal-distal sampling position and age. *J Biomech* 21: 207-212, 1988.

de Boer MD, Maganaris CN, Seynnes OR, Rennie MJ, Narici MV. Time course of muscular, neural and tendinous adaptations to 23 day unilateral lower-limb suspension in young men. *J Physiol* 583: 1079-1091, 2007.

Finni T, Hodgson JA, Lai AM, Edgerton VR, Sinha S. Mapping of movement in the isometrically contracting human soleus muscle reveals details of its structural and functional complexity. *J Appl Physiol* 95: 2128-2133, 2003.

Flint M. Interrelationships of mucopolysaccharide and collagen in connective tissue remodelling. *J Embryol Exp Morphol* 27: 481-495, 1972.

Gans C. Fiber architecture and muscle function. *Exer Sports Sci Rev* 10: 160-207, 1982.

Heinemeier KM, Olesen JL, Haddad F, Schjerling P, Baldwin KM, Kjaer M. Effect of unloading followed by reloading on expression of collagen and related growth factors in rat tendon and muscle. *J Appl Physiol* 106: 178-186, 2009.

Herzog W. Tendon/Aponeurosis. Biomechanics of the Musculo-skeleltal System (eds. Nigg BM and Herzog W). Wiley, England, 146-168, 2007.

Hodgson JA, Finni T, Lai AM, Edgerton VR, Sinha S. Influence of structure on the tissue dynamics of the human soleus muscle observed in MRI studies during isometric contractions. *J Morphol* 267: 584-601, 2006.

Hodgson JA, Shin D, Nagarsekar G, Edgerton VR, Sinha. Amplification of Achilles Tendon Displacement by a Pivot-like Restriction Amplifies Final Displacement of Calcaneous and Rotation of Ankle with Possible Impact on Measured Strain. #6871, Presented at 17th Intl. Soc Mag Res Med Mtng. in Hawaii, 2009.

Hof AL, Van Zandwijk JP, Bobbert MF. Mechanics of human triceps surae muscle in walking, running and jumping. *Acta Physiol Scand* 174: 17-30, 2002.

Hooley CJ, McCrum NG, Cohen RE. The viscoelastic deformation of tendon. J *Biomech* 13: 521-528, 1980.

Iwanuma S, Akagi R, Kurihara T, Ikegawa S, Kanehisa H, Fukunaga T, Kawakami Y. Longitudinal and transverse deformation of human Achilles tendon induced by isometric plantar flexion at different intensities. *J Appl Physiol* 110: 1615-1621, 2011.

Ker RF, Alexander RM, Bennett MB. Why are mammalian tendons so thick? *J Zool* 216: 309–324, 1988.

Kinugasa R, Hodgson JA, Edgerton VR, Shin DD, Sinha S. Reduction in tendon elasticity from unloading is unrelated to its hypertrophy. *J Appl Physiol* 109: 870–877, 2010.

Kinugasa R, Shin D, Yamauchi J, Mishra C, Hodgson JA, Edgerton VR, Sinha S. Phase-contrast MRI reveals mechanical behavior of superficial and deep aponeuroses in human medial gastrocnemius during isometric contraction. *J Appl Physiol* 105: 1312–1320, 2008.

Kotani Y, Cunningham BW, Cappuccino A, Kaneda K, McAfee PC. The effects of spinal fixation and destabilization on the biomechanical and histologic properties of spinal ligaments. An in vivo study. *Spine* 23: 672–683, 1998.

Kubo K, Akima H, Ushiyama J, Tabata I, Fukuoka H, Kanehisa H, Fukunaga T. Effects of 20 days of bed rest on the viscoelastic properties of tendon structures in lower limb muscles. *Br J Sports Med* 38: 324–330, 2004.

Kubo K, Kawakami Y, Kanehisa H, Fukunaga T. Measurement of viscoelastic properties of tendon structures in vivo. *Scand J Med Sci Sports* 12: 3–8, 2002.

Lee HD, Finni T, Hodgson JA, Lai AM, Edgerton VR, Sinha S. Soleus aponeurosis strain distribution following chronic unloading in humans: an in vivo MR phase-contrast study. *J Appl Physiol* 100: 2004–2011, 2006.

Lieber RL, Leonard ME, Brown CG, Trestik CL. Frog semitendinosis tendon load-strain and stress-strain properties during passive loading. *Am J Physiol* 261: C86–92, 1991.

Lieber RL, Leonard ME, Brown-Maupin CG. Effects of muscle contraction on the load-strain properties of frog aponeurosis and tendon. *Cells Tissues Organs* 166: 48–54, 2000.

MacIntyre DL, Eng JJ, Allen TJ. Recovery of lower limb function following 6 weeks of non-weight bearing. *Acta Astronaut* 56: 792–800, 2005.

Maganaris CN, Kawakami Y, Fukunaga T. Changes in aponeurotic dimensions upon muscle shortening: in vivo observations in man. *J Anat* 199: 449–456, 2001.

Maganaris CN, Paul JP. Tensile properties of the in vivo human gastrocnemius tendon. *J Biomech* 35: 1639–1646, 2002.

Maganaris CN, Reeves ND, Rittweger J, Sargeant AJ, Jones DA, Gerrits K, De Haan A. Adaptive response of human tendon to paralysis. *Muscle Nerve* 33: 85–92, 2006.

Maganaris CN, Narici MV, Maffulli N. Biomechanics of the Achilles tendon. *Disabil Rehabil* 30: 1542–1547, 2008.

Matsumoto F, Trudel G, Uhthoff HK, Backman DS. Mechanical effects of immobilization on the Achilles' tendon. *Arch Phys Med Rehabil* 84: 662–667, 2003.

McNeilly CM, Banes AJ, Benjamin M, Ralphs JR. Tendon cells in vivo form a three dimensional network of cell processes linked by gap junctions. *J Anat* 189: 593–600, 1996.

Morgan DL, Proske U, Warren D. Measurements of muscle stiffness and the mechanism of elastic storage of energy in hopping kangaroos. *J Physiol* 282: 253–261, 1978.

Muramatsu T, Muraoka T, Takeshita D, Kawakami Y, Hirano Y, Fukunaga T. Mechanical properties of tendon and aponeurosis of human gastrocnemius muscle in vivo. *J Appl Physiol* 90: 1671–1678, 2001.

Oxorn VM, Agur AM, McKee NH. Resolving discrepancies in image research: the importance of direct observation in the illustration of the human soleus muscle. *J Biocommun* 25: 16–26, 1998.

Paavola M, Kannus P, Jarvinen TA, Khan K, Jozsa L, Jarvinen M. Achilles tendinopathy. *J Bone Joint Surg Am* 84: 2062–2076, 2002.

Patterson-Kane JC, Wilson AM, Firth EC, Parry DA, Goodship AE. Comparison of collagen fibril populations in the superficial digital flexor tendons of exercised and nonexercised thoroughbreds. *Equine Vet J* 29: 121–125, 1997.

Proske U, Morgan DL. Tendon stiffness: methods of measurement and significance for the control of movement. *J Biomech* 20: 75–82, 1987.

Purslow PP. The structure and functional significance of variations in the connective tissue within muscle. *Comp Biochem Physiol A Mol Integr Physiol* 133: 947–966, 2002.

Ralphs JR, Waggett AD, Benjamin M. Actin stress fibres and cell-cell adhesion molecules in tendons: organisation in vivo and response to mechanical loading of tendon cells in vitro. *Matrix Biol* 21: 67–74, 2002.

Reeves ND, Maganaris CN, Ferretti G, Narici MV. Influence of 90-day simulated microgravity on human tendon mechanical properties and the effect of resistive countermeasures. *J Appl Physiol* 98: 2278–2286, 2005.

Reeves NJ, Maganaris CN, Ferretti G, Narici MV. Influence of simulated microgravity on human skeletal muscle architecture and function. *J Gravit Physiol* 9: 153–154, 2002.

Rigby BJ, Hirai N, Spikes JD, Eyring H. The Mechanical Properties of Rat Tail Tendon. *J Gen Physiol* 43: 265–283, 1959.

Rugg SG, Gregor RJ, Mandelbaum BR, Chiu L. *J Biomech* 23: 495–501, 1990.

Schulze K, Gallagher P, Trappe S. Resistance training preserves skeletal muscle function during unloading in humans. *Med Sci Sports Exerc* 34: 303–313, 2002.

Scott SH, Loeb GE. Mechanical properties of aponeurosis and tendon of the cat soleus muscle during whole-muscle isometric contractions. *J Morphol* 224: 73–86, 1995.

Shin D, Finni T, Ahn S, Hodgson JA, Lee HD, Edgerton VR, Sinha S. Effect of chronic unloading and rehabilitation on human Achilles tendon properties: a velocity-encoded phase-contrast MRI study. *J Appl Physiol* 105: 1179–1186, 2008a.

Shin D, Finni T, Ahn S, Hodgson JA, Lee HD, Edgerton VR, Sinha S. In vivo estimation and repeatability of force-length relationship and stiffness of the human achilles tendon using phase contrast MRI. *J Magn Reson Imaging* 28: 1039–1045, 2008b.

Tsuchida T, Yasuda K, Kaneda K, Hayashi K, Yamamoto N, Miyakawa K, Tanaka K. Effects of in situ freezing and stress-shielding on the ultrastructure of rabbit patellar tendons. *J Orthop Res* 15: 904–910, 1997.

Wainwright SD, Biggs WD, Currey JD, Gosline JM. Mechanical design in organisms. Princeton University Press, Princeton, NJ, 88–93, 1982.

Woo SL, Gomez MA, Woo YK, Akeson WH. Mechanical properties of tendons and ligaments. II. The relationships of immobilization and exercise on tissue remodeling. *Biorheology* 19: 397–408, 1982.

Zajac FE. Muscle and tendon: properties, models, scaling, and application to biomechanics and motor control. *Crit Rev Biomed Eng* 17: 359–411, 1989.

Zuurbier CJ, Huijing PA. Influence of muscle geometry on shortening speed of fibre, aponeurosis and muscle. *J Biomech* 25: 1017–1026, 1992.

Part 2

Achilles Tendon Disorders

2

Gene Variants that Predispose to Achilles Tendon Injuries: An Update on Recent Advances

Stuart M. Raleigh[1] and Malcolm Collins[2]
[1]*School of Health, Division of Health and Life Sciences, University of Northampton, Northampton*
[2]*MRC/UCT Research Unit for Exercise Science and Sports Medicine of the South African Medical Research Council and the Department of Human Biology, University of Cape Town, Cape Town*
[1]*UK*
[2]*South Africa*

1. Introduction

There are a number of injuries that affect the Achilles tendon and surrounding tissues. Injuries that affect the surrounding tissues include bursitis and paritendonitis, while Achilles tendinopathy and complete or partial ruptures affect the tendon tissue itself (Puddu, 1976). Although injuries to the Achilles tendon are common as a result of participation in physical activities, Achilles tendon injuries can also occur in sedentary individuals (Young et al., 2005). Although the biological and molecular mechanisms responsible for Achilles tendon injuries are largely unknown, both intrinsic and extrinsic risk factors have nevertheless been implicated in the aetiology of these conditions (Figure 1) (Meeuwisse, 1994; Riley, 2004; September et al., 2006). Genetic susceptibility, which will be the focus of this review, has more recently been included as one of the intrinsic risk factors for chronic Achilles tendinopathy. As illustrated in figure 1, many of the intrinsic risk factors associated with Achilles tendinopathy are in their own right complex phenotypes determined by both genetic and environmental factors. Flexibility (Battie et al., 2008), biological age (Newman et al., 2010), muscle strength (Stewart et al., 2006), weight (Herrera et al., 2010) are all determined by genetic and environmental factors, the development of the male sex on the other hand is determined genetically (Kousta et al., 2010).

A brief summary of the macromolecular structure of tendons is required to understand and review our current knowledge of the genetic basis of Achilles tendon injuries. Tendons have a highly ordered hierarchical structure made up of tightly packed bundles of fibrils consisting predominately of type I collagen fibres (60% of the dry mass of tendons) (Silver et al., 2003). Other quantitively minor collagens, such as type III, V, XIV and XVI collagens form heterotypic fibrils with type I collagen or are associated with the surface of the fibrils

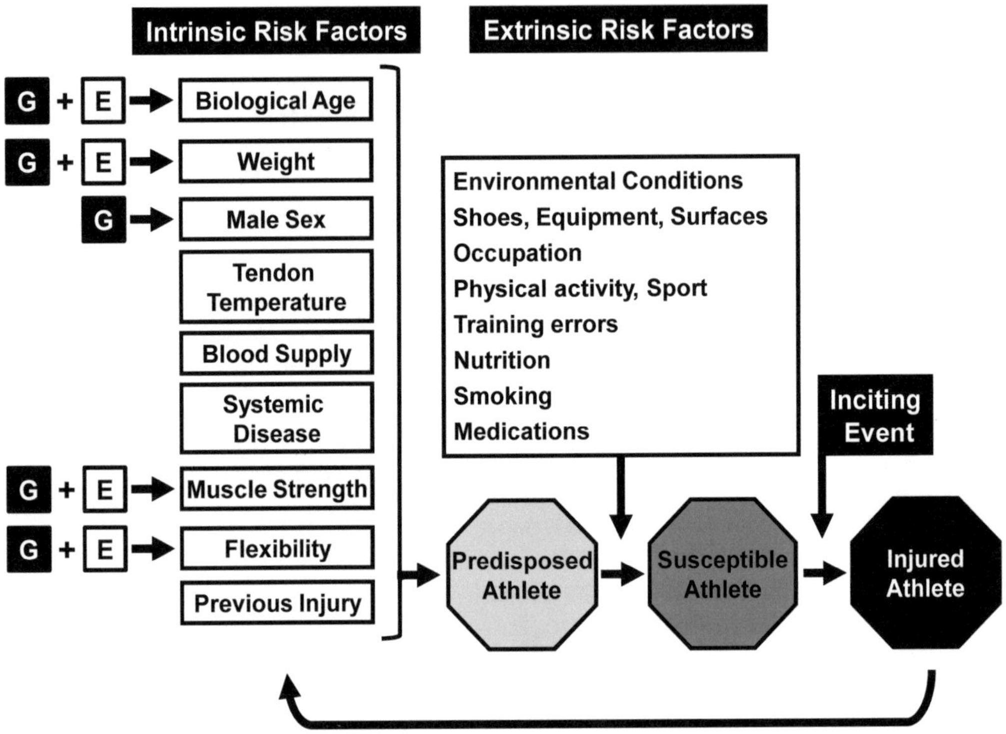

Fig. 1. A diagram illustrating the role of intrinsic and extrinsic risk factors, as well as, the inciting event in the aetiology of Achilles tendon injuries (Meeuwisse, 1994; Riley, 2004; September et al., 2006). Many of the individual intrinsic risk factors are multifactorial phenotypes, which are determined by, to a lesser or greater extent, both genetic (nature, G) and environmental (nurture, E) factors. For acute Achilles tendon injuries the inciting event will be the macrotraumatic event that cause the injury, while the inciting event for a chronic injury will be the point in time when the volume of accumulated micotraumatic damage to the tissue becomes symptomatic. The arrow from the injured Athlete back to list of intrinsic risk factors indicated that once recovered the previous injury predisposes the athlete for additional injuries.

(Canty & Kadler, 2002). These additional collagens play essential roles in tendon biology. Various glycoproteins and proteoglycans, such as tenascin C, decorin, biglycan, aggrecan, lumican, fibromodulin and others, are also important structural components of tendons (Kannus, 2000; Silver, 2003). The expression of many of these protein components has been shown to be altered during tendon injury (Ireland et al., 2001; Alfredson et al., 2003). Many collagen types, cell adhesion molecules, proteoglycans and, matrix metalloproteainases (MMPs), ADAMTS (A Disintegrin And Metalloproteinase with Thrombospondin Motifs - a family of peptidases), tissue inhibitors of metalloproteinases (TIMPS), cell receptors, cytokines and other signalling molecules are either up- or down-regulated in degenerative Achilles tendons (Ireland et al., 2001).

2. Genetic association studies with relevance to injury of the Achilles tendon

Genetic association studies are designed to investigate whether a particular allele or genotype significantly co-segregates with a particular disease trait (Lewis, 2002). Since 2005 such studies have successfully been employed to establish the identity of risk variants for Achilles tendon injuries (Collins & Raleigh, 2009). To date, genetic association studies that are relevant to Achilles tendon injuries have been based on the case-control, candidate gene approach (Collins & Raleigh, 2009). These studies rely on the accurate ascertainment of a clinically distinct phenotype which, as discussed above, can be a challenge for pathology or injury related to the Achilles tendon. In addition to the quality of the phenotypic data the design of a genetic association study must take into account potential confounding factors such as population stratification (Lewis, 2002). For multifactorial conditions such as Achilles tendon injuries other intrinsic factors, such as, amongst others, age and sex, as well as, extrinsic factors, such as type of sporting codes and duration of exposure to high risk activity, should also be considered when selecting cases and controls. The severity of the injury should also be considered when defining the inclusion and exclusion criteria. With respect to chronic Achilles tendinopathy, the following inclusion criteria have previously be used to define a severe phenotype (i) symptoms greater than 6 months, (ii) bilateral Achilles tendinopathy, (iii) multi-injuries, (iv) other tendon injuries and/or (v) early age of initial onset of symptoms (Mokone *et al.* 2005). The selection of appropriately matched controls is as important as the selection of the cases.

For the candidate gene approach, investigators select variants that are plausible *candidates* for a role in the pathology and determine whether an allele or genotype appears at a significantly greater frequency in cases compared to a matched control group (Cordell &, Clayton, 2011). The genome wide approach (GWA) tends to use large numbers of cases and controls that are genotyped for many thousands of tagged single nucleotide polymorphisms (SNPs) (Hosking *et al*, 2011). Investigators predominantly use Affeymetrix or Illumina technology for these investigations but genome wide significance is generally set within the order of $P<0.0000001$ to account for multiple testing (Grant & Hakonarson, 2008). Although GWA studies have clearly advanced our understanding of a number of complex diseases (Grant & Hakonarson, 2008) the technology has not yet been utilised in relation to gene variants that predispose to injuries of the Achilles tendon. In the following section we update our knowledge of gene variants that have been associated with Achilles tendon injuries. Our main focus of this article will be to update the reader on the most recent advances (from 2010 onwards) in the field. However, although we will begin with a brief review of some of the studies that prompted investigators to the search for specific gene variants that could influence the risk of Achilles tendon injuries (section 3) the reader is also advised to consult earlier reviews (September et al. 2006; 2007; Magra and Maffulli, 2007, Collins & Raleigh, 2009).

3. Initial investigations

In 1989 Jozsa and co-workers conducted a retrospective study on the frequency of different blood groups in a Hungarian population that had suffered from tendon ruptures (Jozsa *et al*, 1989). They found an abundance (53%) of blood group O in their cohort compared to 31% of the control sample. The abundance of group O was even higher (69%) in individuals who had sustained a re-rupture (Jozsa *et al*, 1989). Subsequent studies by Kujala and colleagues

(Kujala *et al*, 1992) and Kannus and Natri (Kannus & Natri, 1997 as cited by September, 2007) have documented associations between Achilles tendon rupture and blood group distribution. Interestingly, the relationship between blood group distribution and risk of Achilles tendon rupture was not observed in subsequent work involving 215 Achilles patients recruited in a Finnish cohort (Leppilahti *et al*, 1996), 78 patients in a Scottish based cohort (Maffulli *et al*, 2000) and in a small South African based study involving 75 rupture cases and 131 controls (Mokone, 2006 as cited by September 2007).

Despite the contrasting findings, Mokone and colleagues (Mokone *et al*, 2005) speculated that variants residing in genes encoding tendon structural or regulatory proteins, that were proximal to the ABO chromosome locus (on 9q34) might be candidates for association with Achilles tendon injuries. With this in mind, Mokone and co-workers conducted the first case-control, genetic association study using the candidate gene approach for risk variants relating to Achilles tendon injury. Using a sample of 114 Achilles tendon sufferers and 127 matched controls they established that a dinucleotide repeat polymorphism within the tenascin-C gene (*TNC*), a gene encoding an important enzyme that regulates cell matrix interactions (Jones & Jones, 2000) was associated with Achilles tendon injuries (Mokone *et al*, 2005). Interestingly the study demonstrated that the odds ratios, a quantitative estimate of disease risk based on the carrier of an allele or genotype in cases divided by controls (Lewis et al, 2002), was found to be high. Indeed possession of the 12 and 14 repeat alleles co-segregated with a six fold increase in injury risk (Mokone *et al*, 2005).

Attention was then focused on genomic variation within the gene that encodes the pro-α1(V) chain of collagen type V (*COL5A1*) as a possible susceptibility locus for Achilles tendon injuries. Specifically, using a South African based cohort two polymorphisms were selected within the *COL5A1* gene and one of them (rs12722) was found to significantly associate with chronic Achilles tendinopathy (Mokone *et al*, 2006). The DpnII restriction fragment length polymorphism also investigated by this group was not associated with injury or tendinopathy of the Achilles tendon (Mokone *et al*, 2006). Both these polymorphic markers are located within the 3′-untranslated region (UTR) of the *COL5A1* gene (September *et al*, 2009). Since 2006 confirmation of the association of the rs12722 polymorphism in Achilles tendon pathology has been documented in an Australian population, both as a single marker, and as an inferred haplotype in combination with the C allele of the rs3196378 polymorphism (September *et al*, 2009). In addition to *COL5A1*, three variants within the *MMP3* gene were also found to associate with Achilles tendinopathy in South Africans (Raleigh *et al*, 2009). Interestingly previous (Alfredson *et al*, 2003, Ireland *et al*, 2001) and more recent data (de Mos *et al*, 2009, Jelinsky *et al*, 2011) have shown that MMP3 expression levels are significantly repressed in tissue obtained from Achilles tendinopathic material when compared to controls.

4. Contemporary investigations

Although a diverse group of candidate genes for Achilles tendon injuries were suggested in 2006 (September *et al*, 2006) association studies up to and including 2010 have been limited to variants within genes for proteins involved in the structural or regulatory integrity of tendon or the extracellular matrix (Like *COL5A1* and *MMP3* respectively). To broaden the spectrum of possible candidates, Posthumus and co-workers speculated that members of the transforming growth factor-β (TGF- β) family might influence predisposition to the risk of these injuries (Posthumus *et al*, 2010). They chose this group as logical candidates based on the biochemical functions that TGF-β transcripts had in relation to Achilles tendon function. For example, it was known that TGF-β transfected into healing rabbit Achilles tendon led to enhanced mechanical strength of the tendon due to the regulation of collagen turnover and cross link formation (Hou *et al*, 2006). However, the functional promoter variant rs1800469 of the *TGF-β* gene was not found to co-segregate with Achilles tendon pathology in both South African and Australian Caucasian cohorts (Posthumus *et al*, 2010).

The same investigators then examined the possible role of another variant (rs143383) within a second member of the TGF-β family, namely the growth differentiation factor 5 (*GDF-5*) gene, for association with Achilles tendon injury. They found that carriage of the TT genotype at the rs143383 locus was associated with Achilles tendon pathology in Australian cases and when the data were combined for both cohorts of Australian and South Africans (Posthumus *et al*, 2010). At present a mechanism for how the rs143383 variant exerts its influence on risk of Achilles tendon injury is unknown. However, it is interesting to note that the T allele of this variant has been reported to repress the expression of GDF-5 in tissue obtained from osteoarthritis patients (Egli *et al*, 2009). Furthermore, genotype at this locus (possession of either the T or C allele) has also been shown to govern the binding of the deformed epidermal autoregulatory factor 1 (DEAF-1) transcription factor which may have a role in osteoarthritis susceptibility (Egli *et al*, 2009). Accordingly, genetic variants within the DEAF-1 gene might also be candidates for Achilles tendon injuries. It is also noteworthy that the rs143383 variant has been associated with a range of other musculoskeletal pathologies. For example the rs143383 variant has been shown to be a susceptibility locus for osteoarthritis of the knee (Valdes et al, 2011) and a recent large-scale study in European cohorts has documented that the T allele of rs143383 was associated with lumber disc degeneration in women (F.M Williams *et al*, 2011).

So far we have seen how population-based association studies have enhanced our understanding of the genetic risk factors that can predispose to Achilles tendon injuries. A summary of this data (including only significant associations discussed in sections 3 and 4) is shown in Table 1.

Although studies up to 2010 have focused on single genetic loci or haplotypes that can predispose to Achilles tendon injuries a recent study has utilised a pathway-based model to study predisposing genotypes for Achilles tendon pathology (September et al, 2011). Specifically, the investigators wanted to establish whether allelic variants within a selction of inflammatory genes (interleukin-1β, interleukin-6 and interleukin-1 receptor antagonist), that are differentially expressed in tendinopathy (September *et al*, In Press), were associated with the problem when combined with the *COL5A1* rs12722 variant. Interestingly, they discovered that as single loci none of the variants associated with Achilles tendinopathy. However, in combination, the five variants tested, along with the *COL5A1* variant, were significantly associated ($p<0.005$) with Achilles tendinopathy (September *et al*, 2011). This work demonstrates that polygenic profiling of a complex phenotype like Achilles tendinopathy maybe a superior strategy to use, compared to the single candidate approach, when it comes to understanding the intricate involvement of numerous variants that increase the risk of Achilles tendon problems (September et al, 2011).

Gene	Variant/population	Notes	Reference
Tenascin C (*TNC*)	GT repeat variant within intron 7. South African Caucasian (N=241).	12 and 14 GT repeat variants associated with Achilles tendon injuries. Both allelic and genotypic associations were observed.	Mokone *et al*, 2005
Type V Collagen, α 1 chain, (*COL5A1*)	rs12722 South African Caucasian (N=240).	A2 allele overrepresented in control subjects inferring a protective role for this allele.	Mokone *et al*, 2006
Type V Collagen, α 1 chain, (*COL5A1*)	rs12722 and rs3196378 Australian Caucasian (N=295).	The CC genotype of rs12722 underrepresented in Achilles tendinopathy The rs12722 and rs3196378 variant associated with tendinopathy as an inferred haplotype	September *et al*, 2009
Matrix metalloproteinase 3 (*MMP3*)	rs679620, rs591058 and rs650108 South African Caucasian (N=212).	The GG genotype of rs679620 associated with Achilles tendinopathy. The rs679620, rs591058 and rs650108 variants also associated as an inferred haplotype	Raleigh *et al*, 2009
Growth differentiation factor 5 (GDF-5)	rs143383 Australian and Australian in combination with South African Caucasian (N=406).	The TT genotype of rs143383 overrepresented in Australian and combined Australian and South African	Posthumus *et al*, 2010

Table 1. Genetic variants associated with Achilles tendon pathology in humans. Entries summarise the results of separately published studies investigating a single variant or a haplotype. Information on individual variants can be found by databases hosted by the NCB1 available at http://www.ncbi.nlm.nih.gov/projects/SNP/.

4.1 The *COL5A1* 3'-UTR is functional and associated with other exercise-related phenotypes

Although a genetic association of a sequence variant (rs12722) within the *COL5A1* 3'-UTR has previously been reported for chronic Achilles tendinopathy (Mokone *et al*, 2006; September et al, 2009) in two independent populations, the biological function, if any, of the *COL5A1* 3'-UTR was initially unknown. The 3'-UTR of many eukaryotic protein-coding genes contains regulatory elements, such as miRNA binding sites, involved in the etiology of many diseases (Mazumder et al., 2003). In addition variant rs12722 within the *COL5A1* 3'-UTR is in close proximity with two polymorphic putative miRNA binding sites within the *COL5A1* 3'-UTR (September *et al*, 2009). Due to the structural similarities of tendon and ligaments at the molecular level, the association of the *COL5A1* rs12722 variant with another musculoskeletal soft tissue injury, namely anterior cruciate ligament (ACL) rupture, was investigated. Within females the, CC genotype of SNP rs12722 was significantly under-represented among the cases (Posthumus *et al*, 2009). Although it well document that females are at greater risk for ACL ruptures, the reason for this sex-specific association remains unknown.

Both an increase and decrease in joint range of motion (ROM) is a modifiable risk factor for Achilles tendon injuries (Brown et al., 2011a). In addition, *COL5A1* haploinsufficiency is a common molecular mechanism causing the classic form of Elhers Danlos Syndrome (EDS), which presents with amongst other symptoms joint hypermobility (Malfait et al., 2010). Brown *et al* (2011a) recently reported that the *COL5A1* CC genotype 'protected' individuals against an age-related decline in ROM measurements. Finally the 'less flexible' *COL5A1* TT genotype has been shown to be significantly associated with improved endurance running performance (Posthumus *et al*, 2011; Brown *et al*, 2011b). This finding is in agreement with the published inverse relationship between musculotendineous stiffness and running economy (Arampatzis *et al*, 2006; Dumke *et al*, 2010; Fletcher *et al*, 2010).

As reviewed above the *COL5A1* rs12722 SNP has been associated with Achilles tendinopathy and other exercise-related phenotypes. This single nucleotide DNA sequence variation is not necessarily the cause of these phenotypes. Genetic association studies do not prove cause and effect but highlight genetic regions, proteins or biological pathways that should be further investigated using other biological techniques. This rs12722 SNP is however probably tightly linked to the as yet unknown phenotype-causing polymorphism(s) either within the 3'-UTR of the *COL5A1* gene, other regions of *COL5A1* or a neighboring gene. The results do however indicate that SNP rs12722 is a representative genetic marker for the genetic region (locus) within or surrounding the *COL5A1* gene, which may potentially cause these reported phenotypes.

To test whether the *COL5A1* 3'-UTR was functional, Laguette *et al* (2011) cloned the *COL5A1* 3'-UTR from participants with chronic Achilles tendinopathy or asympomatic controls upstream of a firefly-luciferase reporter gene and transiently transfected the clones into HT1080 cells. They reported an overall increase in COL5A1 mRNA stability in the tendinopathic phenotype and identified two major functional forms of the *COL5A1* 3'-UTR. The one functional form corresponded to the wild type sequence, includes the C allele of SNP rs12722, and was identified in most of the clones generated from asymptomatic controls. The second functional form, on the other hand, included the T allele of SNP rs12722 and was predominantly identified in the Achilles tendinopathic patients. An overall increase in mRNA stability was asscoiated with the second functional form of the COL5A1 3′-UTR, which was cloned from participants with chronic Achilles tendinopathy (Laguette *et al*, 2011).

The *COL5A1* gene encodes the α1 chain of type V. Although present in much smaller amounts than type I collagen, type V collagen plays a critical role in the regulation of type I collagen fibril assembly and lateral growth (fibrillogenesis) (Wenstrup *et al*, 2011). There is an inverse relationship between fibril diameter and type V collagen content, increased type V collagen content in the fibril causes thinner fibres. This in turn is believed to alter the mechanical properties of tissues such as the Achilles tendon (Collins & Posthumus, In Press). Type V collagen is therefore an important structural component of tendons and other connective tissues. In addition, since both copies of the *COL5A1* gene are required for normal collagen fibril formation (Wenstrup *et al*, 2006; Malfait *et al*, 2010), it is possible that relatively small changes in *COL5A1* mRNA stability within the normal physiological range (non-pathological) could result in inter-individual variation in fibrillogenesis, mechanical properties and susceptibility to musculoskeletal soft tissue injuries, as well as, variations in flexibility and endurance running performance (Collins & Posthumus, In Press).

4.2 Fibrilogenesis and Achilles injuries

As described above a variant within the functional 3′-UTR of *COL5A1* is associated with chronic Achilles tendinopathy, another musculoskeletal soft tissue injury and other exercise related phenotypes. In addition we have mentioned that type V collagen is essential for life and is an important protein regulating fibrillogenesis in tendons and other connective tissues. Other proteins besides type V collagen also regulate fibrillogenesis and therefore the gene encoding these proteins should also be considered ideal candidate genes for chronic Achilles tendinopathy.

Other proteins involved in fibrillogenesis, including type XI, XII and XIV collagens, the proteoglycans, decorin, lumican and fibromodulin, as well as the matricellular protein, thrombospondin 2 (Fichard *et al*, 1995; Reed & Iozzo, 2002; Chakravarti, 2002; Bornstein *et al*, 2000). In addition, like tenascin C which is regulated in tendons by mechanical stress, type XII and type XIV collagens are also expressed in both tendons and ligaments and regulated by mechanical stretch (Chiquet, 1999; Nishiyama *et al*, 1994). It has also been postulated that type XII and XIV collagens play an important role in the regulation of fibril assembly due to their ability to interact with proteoglycans such as decorin, lumican and fibromodulin (Ezura *et al*, 2000; Svensson *et al*, 2000; Danielson *et al*, 1997). Immunoelectron microscopy has shown that both these collagen types are associated with the surface of collagen fibrils, suggesting that they might possible be able to form interfibrillar connections and mediate fibril interaction with other extracellular and cell surface molecules (Schuppan *et al*, 1990; Keene *et al* 1991; Zhang *et al*, 1993; Walchli *et al*, 1994). Both type XII and XIV collagens are homotrimers and belong to the sub-family of fibril-associated collagens with interrupted triple helices (FACIT) and are encoded for by the *COL12A1* and *COL14A1* genes, respectively (Shaw & Olsen, 1991; Mayne & Brewton, 1993; Olsen, 1995). Variants within *COL12A1* and *COL14A1* were however not associated with these injuries (September *et al*, 2008). Although some of the tested variants were non-synonymous (changed an amino acid in the protein), we cannot exclude the possibility that other untested variants within

COL12A1 and *COL14A1* are associated with Achilles tendinopathy. Interestingly the variants within the *COL12A1* gene were however associated with ACL ruptures in females (Posthumus *et al*, 2010). The association of other genes encoding for proteins involved in fibrillogenesis remains to be tested.

5. Future research, applied and clinical significance

Several genetic markers located within genes encoding for tendon structural proteins, extracellular proteinases and signaling molecules have been shown to be associated with chronic Achilles tendinopathy. These results indicate that the genetic contribution for these injuries is polygenic and that several biological pathways are involved. The polygenic natures of Achilles tendon injuries is not surprising, since, as illustrated in figure 1, many of the intrinsic risk factors are determined by both genetic and environmental factors.

Most of the reported associations have been confirmed in a second population (September et al, 2009; Posthumus *et al*, 2010). The sample sizes of the study population have however generally been small and therefore such studies should be repeated in other populations as well as non-Caucasian populations. The association of these variants should also be tested in Achilles tendon ruptures. Interestingly, the preliminary findings suggest that there might be similarities and differences when identifying genetic elements associated within ruptures and tendinopathy (e.g. Mokone *et al*, 2005; 2006).

Although human DNA is over 99.9% identical (Burton et al., 2011), the 0.1% sequence differences (polymorphisms) partially explains why (i) every athlete is not identical (biological variation), (ii) every athlete's Achilles tendon structure is not identical, (iii) the tendons response to loading is not identical, and (iv) their response to healing (treatment modalities) is not identical. As previously discussed in an editorial (Collins, 2010), these factors fall within the developing disciple of personalized medicine. With this in mind, genetic markers could one day be included in multifactorial models to explain inter-individual variation in susceptibility to injury, as well as, response to training, prevention programmes, treatment and rehabilitation. Much more work is however required before this becomes a reality. It is however important to reiterate that Achilles tendon and other musculoskeletal soft tissue injuries are all multifactorial in nature. There is no single factor that causes any of these injuries. The inclusion of genetic markers into any model that has clinical applications could never be used for diagnostic purposes. Their inclusion will only help in determining risk. The inclusion of genetic risk factors in risk models raises ethical issues, which need to be addressed before any clinical service becomes a reality (Collins, 2010; A.G Williams & Wackerhage, 2009).

Besides the obvious clinical applications, the identification of genetic elements associated with Achilles tendon injuries will compliment the other biological disciplines in understanding and elucidating the biological mechanisms of these injuries. This is a less discussed and appreciated application. It is however currently an important application of this area of research. Some of the previously reported associated genetic markers are functional. It is therefore possible to postulate how these genes, or more specifically their protein products are involved in the etiology of the injuries. These possible mechanism need to be proved or verified using other biological techniques. As previously reviewed (Collins

& Posthumus, In Press) work is currently ongoing to explain how variants within the 3'-UTR of the *COL5A1* gene could be directly involved in the susceptibility to Achilles tendon injuries. One of the reasons the current risk models (figure 1) have limited practical application in determining risk of injury for a individual athlete is that they are not based on an understanding on the biological mechanisms causing the injury.

We propose that future risk models should be developed around an understanding of the biological mechanisms of Achilles tendon injuries (Figure 2). Current and future research using human molecular genetics and other biological techniques will play an important part in elucidating the mechanisms and developing more appropriate risk models.

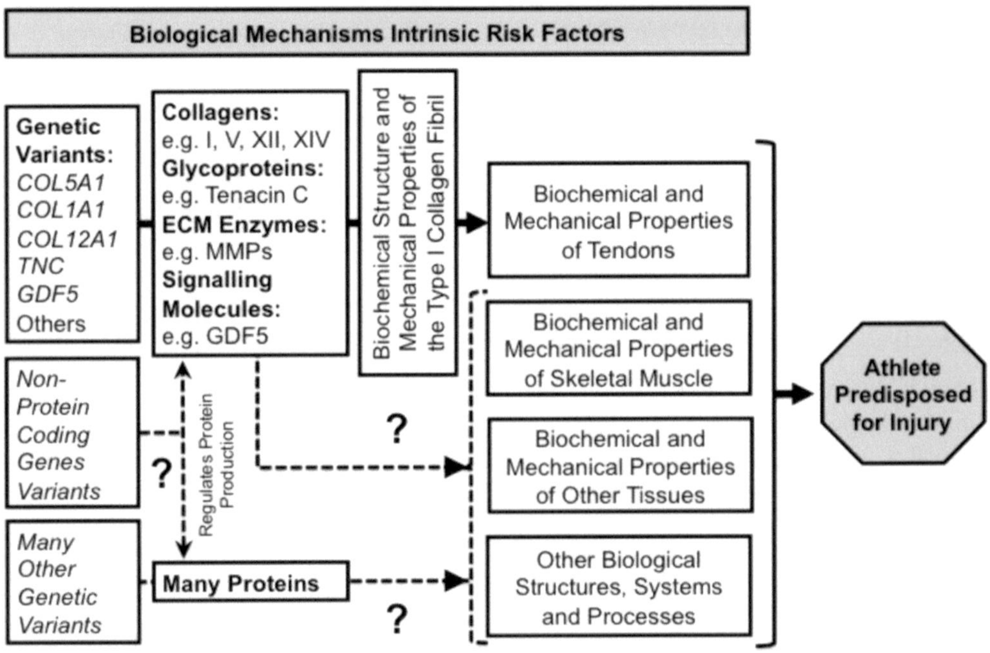

Fig. 2. A schematic illustrating how proposed molecular and biological mechanisms could more accurately describe intrinsic component for Achilles tendon injury risk. In this hypothetical model, inter-individual variations in the biochemical and mechanical properties of the tendon, skeletal muscle and other tissues, as well as, other biological structures, systems and processes cause susceptibility to Achilles tendon injuries. Structural differences and levels of proteins within the tissue cause the inter-individual variations. These differences are in turn partly determined by functional genetic variations within protein-coding and non-coding genes. The predisposed athletes will become a susceptible athlete if exposed to the appropriate extrinsic factors and only become injured (acute injury) or symptomatic (overuse injury) after a specific, usually identifiable, inciting event as illustrated in figure 1.

6. References

Alfredson H, Lorentzon, M., Bäckman, S., Bäckman, A., & Lerner, U. H. (2003). cDNA-arrays and real-time quantitative PCR techniques in the investigation of chronic Achilles tendinosis. *Journal of orthopaedic research*: official publication of the Orthopaedic Research Society, 21(6), 970–975.

Arampatzis A, De Monte, G., Karamanidis, K., Morey-Klapsing, G., Stafilidis, S., & Brüggemann, G.-P. (2006). Influence of the muscle-tendon unit's mechanical and morphological properties on running economy. *The Journal of experimental biology*, 209(Pt 17), 3345–3357.

Battie MC LE, Videman T, Burton K, Kaprio J. (2008).Heritability of lumbar flexibility and the role of disc degeneration and body weight. *Journal of Applied Physiology*, 104: 379-385.

Bornstein P, Armstrong, L. C., Hankenson, K. D., Kyriakides, T. R., & Yang, Z. (2000). Thrombospondin 2, a matricellular protein with diverse functions. *Matrix biology : journal of the International Society for Matrix Biology*, 19(7), 557–568.

Brown JC, Miller, C.-J., Schwellnus, M. P., & Collins, M. (2011a). Range of motion measurements diverge with increasing age for COL5A1 genotypes. *Scandinavian Journal of Medicine & Science in Sports. In press*

Brown JC, Miller, C.-J., Posthumus, M., Schwellnus, M. P., & Collins, M. (2011b). The *COL5A1* gene, ultra-marathon running performance and range of motion. An original investigation. *International Journal of Sports Physiology and Performance. In Press*

Burton PR, Tobin MD Hopper JL (2011). Genetic association studies, In: *An introduction to genetic epidemiology*, Edited by Palmer LJ, Burton PR and Davey Smith, G, (5-38), The Policy press, ISBN 9781861348975, Bristol, UK

Canty EG, & Kadler, K. E. (2002). Collagen fibril biosynthesis in tendon: a review and recent insights. *Comparative biochemistry and physiology Part A, Molecular & integrative physiology*, 133(4), 979–985.

Chakravarti S. Functions of lumican and fibromodulin: lessons from knockout mice. *Glycoconjugate Journal*, 19: 287-293, 2002.

Chiquet, M. (1999). Regulation of extracellular matrix gene expression by mechanical stress. *Matrix biology : journal of the International Society for Matrix Biology*, 18(5), 417–426.

Collins M. (2010). Genetic risk factors for soft-tissue injuries 101: a practical summary to help clinicians understand the role of genetics and 'personalised medicine'. *British Journal of Sports Medicine* 44: 915-917.

Collins M, and Posthumus M. (2011) Type V Collagen Genotype and Exercise-Related Phenotype Relationships: A Novel Hypothesis. *Exercise and Sports Sciences Reviews. In press*

Collins M, and Raleigh SM. (2009). Genetic risk factors for musculoskeletal soft tissue injuries. *Medicine Sport Science*54: 136-149.

Cordell HJ, and Clayton DG (2011). Genetic association studies, In: *An introduction to genetic epidemiology*, Edited by Palmer LJ, Burton PR and Davey Smith, G, (61-89), The Policy press, ISBN 9781861348975, Bristol, UK

Danielson KG, Baribault, H., Holmes, D. F., Graham, H., Kadler, K. E., & Iozzo, R. V. (1997). Targeted disruption of decorin leads to abnormal collagen fibril morphology and skin fragility. *The Journal of cell biology*, 136(3), 729–743.

de Mos M, Joosten LA, Oppers-Walgreen B, van Schie JT, Jahr H, van Osch GJ, and Verhaar JA. (2009). Tendon degeneration is not mediated by regulation of Toll-like receptors 2 and 4 in human tenocytes. *Journal of Orthopaedic Research*27: 1043-1047.

Dumke CL, Pfaffenroth, C. M., McBride, J. M., & McCauley, G. O. (2010). Relationship between muscle strength, power and stiffness and running economy in trained male runners. *International journal of sports physiology and performance*, 5(2), 249–261.

Egli RJ, Southam L, Wilkins JM, Lorenzen I, Pombo-Suarez M, Gonzalez A, Carr A, Chapman K, and Loughlin J. (2009). Functional analysis of the osteoarthritis susceptibility-associated GDF5 regulatory polymorphism. *Arthritis & Rheumatism* 60: 2055-2064.

Ezura Y, Chakravarti, S., Oldberg, A., Chervoneva, I., & Birk, D. E. (2000). Differential expression of lumican and fibromodulin regulate collagen fibrillogenesis in developing mouse tendons. *The Journal of cell biology*, 151(4), 779–788.

Fichard A, Kleman, J. P., & Ruggiero, F. (1995). Another look at collagen V and XI molecules. *Matrix biology : journal of the International Society for Matrix Biology*, 14(7), 515–531.

Fletcher JR, Esau SP, and MacIntosh BR. (2010) Changes in tendon stiffness and running economy in highly trained distance runners. *European Journal of Applied Physiology*110: 1037-1046.

Grant SF, and Hakonarson H. (2008). Microarray technology and applications in the arena of genome-wide association. *Clinical Chemistry*54: 1116-1124.

Herrera BM, & Lindgren, C. M. (2010). The genetics of obesity. *Current diabetes reports*, 10(6), 498–505.

Hosking FJ, Dobbins SE, and Houlston RS. (2011). Genome-wide association studies for detecting cancer susceptibility. *British Medical Bulletin*, 97: 27-46.

Hou Y, Mao Z, Wei X, Lin L, Chen L, Wang H, Fu X, Zhang J, and Yu C. (2009). The roles of TGF-beta1 gene transfer on collagen formation during Achilles tendon healing. *Biochemical and biophysical research communications*, 383: 235-239.

Ireland D, Harrall, R., Curry, V., Holloway, G., Hackney, R., Hazleman, B., & Riley, G. (2001). Multiple changes in gene expression in chronic human Achilles tendinopathy. *Matrix biology : journal of the International Society for Matrix Biology*, 20(3), 159–169.

Jelinsky SA, Rodeo SA, Li J, Gulotta LV, Archambault JM, and Seeherman HJ. (2011). Regulation of gene expression in human tendinopathy. *BMC Musculoskeletal Disorders* 12: 86.

Jones FS, and Jones PL. (2000). The tenascin family of ECM glycoproteins: structure, function, and regulation during embryonic development and tissue remodeling. *Developmental Dynamics* 218: 235-259.

Jozsa L, Balint JB, Kannus P, Reffy A, and Barzo M. (1989). Distribution of blood groups in patients with tendon rupture. An analysis of 832 cases. The Journal of bone and oint surgery. British volume, 71: 272-274.

Kannus P. (2000). Structure of the tendon connective tissue. *Scandinavian journal of medicine & science in sports*,10: 312-320,

Kannus P, and Natri A. (1997). Etiology and pathophysiology of tendon ruptures in sports. *Scandinavian journal of medicine & science in sports,*7: 107-112.

Keene DR, Lunstrum, G. P., Morris, N. P., Stoddard, D. W., & Burgeson, R. E. (1991). Two type XII-like collagens localize to the surface of banded collagen fibrils *The Journal of cell biology*, 113(4), 971–978.

Kousta E, Papathanasiou, A., & Skordis, N. (2010). Sex determination and disorders of sex development according to the revised nomenclature and classification in 46,XX individuals *Hormones (Athens, Greece)*, 9(3), 218–131.

Kujala UM, Jarvinen M, Natri A, Lehto M, Nelimarkka O, Hurme M, Virta L, and Finne J. (1992). ABO blood groups and musculoskeletal injuries. *Injury* 23: 131-133,

Laguette M-J, Abrahams, Y., Prince, S., & Collins, M. (2011). Sequence variants within the 3'-UTR of the COL5A1 gene alters mRNA stability: Implications for musculoskeletal soft tissue injuries *Matrix biology : journal of the International Society for Matrix Biology*, 30(5-6), 338–345.

Leppilahti J, Puranen J, and Orava S. (1996). ABO blood group and Achilles tendon rupture. *Annales chirurgiae et gynaecologiae,* 85: 369-371.

Lewis CM. (2002). Genetic association studies: design, analysis and interpretation. *Briefings in bioinformatics,* 3: 146-153.

Maffulli N, Reaper JA, Waterston SW, and Ahya T. (2000). ABO blood groups and achilles tendon rupture in the Grampian Region of Scotland. *Clinical journal of sport medicine : official journal of the Canadian Academy of Sport Medicine,* 10: 269-271.

Magra M and Maffulli N. (2007). Genetics: Does it play a role in tendinopathy?. Clinical Journal of Sports Medicine 17 (4), 231-233.

Malfait F, Wenstrup, R. J., & De Paepe, A. (2010). Clinical and genetic aspects of Ehlers-Danlos syndrome, classic type. *Genetics in medicine : official journal of the American College of Medical Genetics*, 12(10), 597–605.

Mayne R, and Brewton RG. (1993). New members of the collagen superfamily. *Current opinion in cell biology,* 5: 883-890.

Mazumder B, Seshadri, V., & Fox, P. L. (2003). Translational control by the 3'-UTR: the ends specify the means. *Trends in Biochemical Sciences*, 28(2), 91–98.

Meeuwisse WH. (1994). Assessing causation in sport injury: a multifactorial model. Clinical journal of sport medicine : official journal of the Canadian Academy of Sport Medicine, 4:166–170.

Mokone GG, Schwellnus, M. P., Noakes, T. D., & Collins, M. (2006). The COL5A1 gene and Achilles tendon pathology. *Scandinavian Journal of Medicine & Science in Sports*, 16(1), 19–26.

Mokone GG, Gajjar, M., September, A. V., Schwellnus, M. P., Greenberg, J., Noakes, T. D., & Collins, M. (2005). The guanine-thymine dinucleotide repeat polymorphism within the tenascin-C gene is associated with achilles tendon injuries. *The American Journal of Sports Medicine*, 33(7), 1016–1021.

Newman AB, Walter, S., Lunetta, K. L., Garcia, M. E., Slagboom, P. E., Christensen, K., Arnold, A. M., et al. (2010). A meta-analysis of four genome-wide association studies of survival to age 90 years or older: the Cohorts for Heart and Aging

Research in Genomic Epidemiology Consortium *The journals of gerontology Series A, Biological sciences and medical sciences*, 65(5), 478–487.

Nishiyama T, McDonough AM, Bruns RR, and Burgeson RE. (1994). Type XII and XIV collagens mediate interactions between banded collagen fibers in vitro and may modulate extracellular matrix deformability. The *Journal of Biological Chemistry*, 269: 28193-28199

Olsen BR. (1995). New insights into the function of collagens from genetic analysis. *Current opinion in cell biology* 7: 720-727.

Posthumus M, September, A. V., O'cuinneagain, D., van der Merwe, W., Schwellnus, M. P., & Collins, M. (2009). The COL5A1 gene is associated with increased risk of anterior cruciate ligament ruptures in female participants. *The American Journal of Sports Medicine*, 37(11), 2234–2240.

Posthumus M, Schwellnus, M. P., & Collins, M. (2011). The COL5A1 gene: a novel marker of endurance running performance. *Medicine and science in sports and exercise*, 43(4), 584–589.

Posthumus M, September, A. V., O'cuinneagain, D., van der Merwe, W., Schwellnus, M. P., & Collins, M. (2010). The association between the COL12A1 gene and anterior cruciate ligament ruptures. *British Journal of Sports Medicine*, 44(16), 1160–1165.

Posthumus M, Collins M, Cook J, Handley CJ, Ribbans WJ, Smith RK, Schwellnus MP, and Raleigh SM. (2010). Components of the transforming growth factor-beta family and the pathogenesis of human Achilles tendon pathology--a genetic association study. *Rheumatology (Oxford)* 49: 2090-2097.

Puddu G, Ippolito, E., & Postacchini, F. (1976). A classification of Achilles tendon disease. *The American Journal of Sports Medicine*, 4(4), 145–150.

Raleigh SM, van der Merwe L, Ribbans WJ, Smith RK, Schwellnus MP, and Collins M. (2009). Variants within the MMP3 gene are associated with Achilles tendinopathy: possible interaction with the COL5A1 gene. *British Journal of Sports Medicine* 43: 514-520,

Reed CC, & Iozzo, R. V. (2002). The role of decorin in collagen fibrillogenesis and skin homeostasis. *Glycoconjugate journal*, 19(4-5), 249–255.

Riley, G. (2004). The pathogenesis of tendinopathy. A molecular perspective. *Rheumatology (Oxford, England)*, 43(2), 131–142.

Schuppan D, Cantaluppi, M. C., Becker, J., Veit, A., Bunte, T., Troyer, D., Schuppan, F., et al. (1990). Undulin, an extracellular matrix glycoprotein associated with collagen fibrils. *The Journal of biological chemistry*, 265(15), 8823–8832.

September AV, Cook, J., Handley, C. J., Van Der Merwe, L., Schwellnus, M. P., & Collins, M. (2009). Variants within the COL5A1 gene are associated with Achilles tendinopathy in two populations. *British Journal of Sports Medicine*, 43(5), 357–365.

September AV, Mokone, G. G., Schwellnus, M. P., & Collins, M. (2006). Genetic risk factors for Achilles tendon injuries. *International SportMed Journal*, 7(3), 201–215.

September AV, Posthumus, M., Van Der Merwe, L., Schwellnus, M. P., Noakes, T. D., & Collins, M. (2008). The COL12A1 and COL14A1 genes and Achilles tendon injuries. *International journal of sports medicine*, 29(3), 257–263.

September AV, Schwellnus, M. P., & Collins, M. (2007). Tendon and ligament injuries: the genetic component. *British Journal of Sports Medicine*, 41(4), 241–246.

September AV, Nell EM, O'Connell K, Cook J, Handley CJ, van der Merwe L, Schwellnus M, and Collins M. (2011). A pathway-based approach investigating the genes encoding interleukin-1{beta}, interleukin-6 and the interleukin-1 receptor antagonist provides new insight into the genetic susceptibility of Achilles tendinopathy. *British Journal of Sports Medicine. In Press*

Shaw LM, and Olsen BR. (1991). FACIT collagens: diverse molecular bridges in extracellular matrices. *Trends in Biochemical Sciences,* 16: 191-194.

Silver FH, Freeman, J. W., & Seehra, G. P. (2003). Collagen self-assembly and the development of tendon mechanical properties. *Journal of Biomechanics,* 36(10), 1529–1553.

Stewart CEH, & Rittweger, J. (2006). Adaptive processes in skeletal muscle: molecular regulators and genetic influences. *Journal of musculoskeletal & neuronal interactions,* 6(1), 73–86.

Svensson L, Närlid, I., & Oldberg, A. (2000). Fibromodulin and lumican bind to the same region on collagen type I fibrils. *FEBS letters*, 470(2), 178–182.

Valdes AM, Evangelou E, Kerkhof HJ, Tamm A, Doherty SA, Kisand K, Kerna I, Uitterlinden A, Hofman A, Rivadeneira F, Cooper C, Dennison EM, Zhang W, Muir KR, Ioannidis JP, Wheeler M, Maciewicz RA, van Meurs JB, Arden NK, Spector TD, and Doherty M. (2011) The GDF5 rs143383 polymorphism is associated with osteoarthritis of the knee with genome-wide statistical significance. *Annals of the rheumatic diseases,* 70: 873-875.

Wälchli C, Koch, M., Chiquet, M., Odermatt, B. F., & Trueb, B. (1994). Tissue-specific expression of the fibril-associated collagens XII and XIV. *Journal of Cell Science,* 107 (Pt 2), 669–681.

Wenstrup RJ, Smith, S. M., Florer, J. B., Zhang, G., Beason, D. P., Seegmiller, R. E., Soslowsky, L. J and Birk DE. (2011). Regulation of collagen fibril nucleation and initial fibril assembly involves coordinate interactions with collagens V and XI In developing tendon. *The Journal of Biological Chemistry,* 286, 20455-20465

Wenstrup RJ, Florer, J. B., Davidson, J. M., Phillips, C. L., Pfeiffer, B. J., Menezes, D. W., Chervoneva, I and Birk DE. (2006). Murine model of the Ehlers-Danlos syndrome. col5a1 haploinsufficiency disrupts collagen fibril assembly at multiple stages. *The Journal of biological chemistry,* 281(18), 12888–12895.

Williams AG, and Wackerhage H. Genetic testing of athletes. *Medicine Sport Science,* 54: 176-186, 2009.

Williams FM, Popham M, Hart DJ, de Schepper E, Bierma-Zeinstra S, Hofman A, Uitterlinden AG, Arden NK, Cooper C, Spector TD, Valdes AM, and van Meurs J. (2011). GDF5 single-nucleotide polymorphism rs143383 is associated with lumbar disc degeneration in Northern European women. *Arthritis and rheumatism,* 63: 708-712.

Young JS, Kumta SM, and Maffulli N. (2005) Achilles tendon rupture and tendinopathy: management of complications. *Foot and ankle clinics,* 10: 371-382.

Zhang X, Schuppan D, Becker J, Reichart P, and Gelderblom HR. (1993). Distribution of undulin, tenascin, and fibronectin in the human periodontal ligament and cementum: comparative immunoelectron microscopy with ultra-thin cryosections. *The journal of histochemistry and cytochemistry: official journal of the Histochemistry Society* 41: 245-251.

Part 3

Achilles Tendon Tendinopathies

3

Tendon Healing with Growth Factors

Sebastian Müller, Atanas Todorov,
Patricia Heisterbach and Martin Majewski
University of Basel,
Department of Orthopaedic Surgery and Traumatology
Switzerland

1. Introduction

The incidence of sport injuries has increased in recent years due to fitness training and growing participation in sport activities by the general public. The tendon rupture was regarded as an injury typical of high-performance athletes. As physical and recreational activities become more and more popular followed by an increased frequency of soft tissue injuries, health care costs are raising. Tendon lacerations, ruptures, or inflammation cause marked morbidity and has a major impact on work, recreational activities, and daily needs. Tendon ruptures and tears are slow healing injuries that are often treated surgically with unsatisfactory results for some patients. As biology of healing processes and the influence of growth factors are becoming more and more clear, one can consider introducing biological therapy into clinical use. For optimizing treatment more understanding is needed. Therefore tendon physiology, pathology, ruptures biology and functionality, normal healing process, as well as the role of polypeptide factors during healing need to be known.

The injury itself initiates several pathways of signalling that recruits fibroblasts and stimulates tenocytes for collagen synthesis and other extracellular components. Together with some mechanical stress, the healing process is able to restore tendon tissue partially or sometimes close-to-normal. However, repaired tendon tissue rarely achieves functional normal tendon. To improve such results, this complex process requires a combination of treatments as: non-operative or operative treatment to restore length, early functional therapy for mechanical stimulation, and tissue engineering to provide additional growth factors.

These treatment modalities may improve tissue healing, tendon gliding, mechanical strength, and return to normal function while preventing tendon gapping, ruptures, and extensive adhesions. Recent advances in bioengineering including the use of growth factors, mesenchymal stem cells and biocompatible scaffolds are promising.

Although the effect of growth factors on tendon healing is impressive, it has become increasingly clear that tendon repair is not triggered by a single growth factor but requires the interplay of various such factors. Collectively, they exert powerful and comprehensive effects on healing. Therefore further research is needed.

2. Tendon structure and healing

2.1 Tendon structure

Tendons functionally connect the dynamic and static components of the locomotive apparatus. Disturbances in the propagation of force from muscle to bone are associated with a considerable loss of function of the extremity. In order to fulfill these functions tendons have special morphological characteristics: fibers are closely packed in a parallel arrangement. The high collagen content and the parallel orientation of the fibers give them extraordinary tensile strength, the highest of any tissue in the body. This characteristic results, for the most part, from the composition and structure of the collagen and elastic fibers, and their interplay. Collagen accounts for 70% of the dry weight of tendons, 95% of which is collagen type I and to a smaller extent elastin (Birk & Trelstad, 1984; Molloy et al., 2003). The remaining 5% is composed of collagen type III as well as a glycosaminoglycan component of approximately 0.5% (Ducy & Karsenty, 2003; Gerich et al., 1996). Collagen is rich in proline and glycine and contains hydroxyproline and hydroxylysine. Lysine and proline residues get hydroxylated within fibroblasts. Hydroxyproline and hydroxylysine are important in maintaining tendon structure; they form H-bridges and hydroxylysine residues are involved in the covalent cross-linking of collagen fibers (Molloy et al., 2003). The individual collagen fibers are arranged in fascicles that contain nerve fibers, blood and lymph vessels (Petersen et al., 2003a; Petersen et al., 2004). Within the fascicles there exist specialized fibroblasts called tenocytes, which exhibit a high degree of organization. Vertically they appear star-like and longitudinally they appear to be arranged in a row along the fibers. This special orientation of the cells reflects their function. These cells are capable of synthesizing fibrillose as well as non-fibrillar components of the extracellular matrix and can also resorb collagen fibers (Chan et al., 1997; Gerich et al., 1996). The fascicles are covered with epitenon, which in turn is covered with paratenon. A fluid film lies between these two layers, which make the movements of the tendon possible.

2.2 Tendon healing

Study of the physiology of tendon healing has revealed two mechanisms of healing, intrinsic and extrinsic healing (Grotendorst, 1988; Hefti & Stoll 1995). During intrinsic healing the tendon with the surrounding tendon sheath are obliterated. The healing of defects between the tendon ends consists of an exudative and a formative phase which are for the most part similar to wound healing in other parts of the body (Maffulli et al., 2000). The concept of extrinsic tendon healing is based on the fact that the cells responsible for the process migrate from the peripheral tendon sheath to the area of the defect (Özkan et al., 1999). This was seen in animal experiments, where fibroblasts and newly formed collagen fibers in the first days after the injury were arranged in a radial manner and then after several days oriented in a longitudinal fashion according to the stress load profile of the tendon. It is now assumed that both extrinsic and intrinsic tendon healing play important roles. Tendon healing can be summarized as follows (Gerich et al., 1996).

2.3 The three phases of tendon healing

Tendon healing occurs in three phases, an inflammatory, a repair, and a remodeling phase (Lou et al., 1996). The inflammatory phase occurs during the first three to five days after injury. It is characterized by the migration and proliferation of cells from the extrinsic peritendonal tissue such as the paratenon, subcutaneous fat tissue and fascia and the intrinsic epitenon and endotenon (Party et al., 1978). At first the extrinsic tissue repair predominates. In this manner the tissue defect is filled with granulation tissue of extrinsic origin. The fibroblasts, which migrate into the area of the injury, have phagocytic properties and at first are found in a radiating pattern along the length of the tendon. During this inflammatory phase the defect zone is filled with tissue that includes parts of the ruptured tendon and hematoma and the biomechanical stability is dependent on the fibrin fibers (Lou et al., 1996).

Around the fifth day the fibroblasts, which have migrated into the wound area, start to synthesize collagen. Initially there is no uniform orientation of the newly formed collagen fibers. They contribute to a great degree to the biomechanical stability of the defect zone. Fibroblasts are the dominant cell type within the lesion and the collagen component increases continuously until the fifth week.

In the fourth week increased proliferation of fibroblasts of intrinsic origin occurs. These fibroblasts are mostly derived from the endotenon and actively remodel collagen. As tissue maturation proceeds collagen fibers increasingly orient themselves along the functional stress axis of the tendon. This reparative phase takes place approximately two months after injury.

Time (days)	Phase	Process
0	**Immediately post-injury**	Clot formation around the wound
0-1	**Inflammatory**	First battery of growth factors and inflammatory molecules produced by cells within the blood clot
1-2		Invasion by extrinsic cells, phagocytosis
2-4	**Proliferation**	Further invasion by extrinsic cells, followed by a second battery of growth factors that stimulate fibroblast proliferation
4-7	**Reparative**	Collagen deposition; granulation tissue formation; revascularisation
7-14		Injury site becomes more organised; extracellular matrix is produced in large amounts
14-21	**Remodelling**	Decreases in cellular and vascular content; increases in collagen type I
21+		Collagen continues to become more organised and cross-linked with healthy matrix outside the injury area. Collagen ratios, water content and cellularity begin to approach normal levels

Table 1. Summary of the healing process in tendons and ligaments. From Molloy et al., 2003.

Final biomechanical stability is achieved in response to resuming normal movement. During this period further organization of the collagen fibers along the stress axis of the tendon occurs. In addition, tensile strength is increased through cross-linking between the collagen fibrils. There is a shift from the synthesis of type III collagen to the mechanically more stable type I collagen (Möller et al., 1998; Pierce et al., 1995). There is no complete regeneration of the tendon lesion in spite of the intensive remodeling in the initial months after injury. The repaired tissue remains hypercellular and there is a shift in favor of thinner collagen fibrils, which compromises its biomechanical characteristics (Maffulli et al., 2002; Möller et al., 1998). In the flexor tendon, an increased production of type III collagen is seen up to 14 months after injury (Pierce et al., 1995). These results are mirrored in a reduced collagen fibrillar diameter, which is seen after tendon injury (Janqueira et al., 1978; Möller et al., 1998). The concentration of collagen type III with this type of regenerate is inversely proportional with the mechanical resilience of the healed tendon (Laemmli, 1970).

Collagen type analyses performed after Achilles tendon rupture indicate a decrease in collagen type I alongside a significant increase in the amount of collagen type III (Ducy & Karsenty, 2003). An elevation of the amount of collagen type III is thought to be the cause of reduced tensile strength in connective tissue due to the reduced cross-linking of this collagen type (Janqueira et al., 1978, Jozsa et al., 1984; Lou et al., 1997, Maffulli et al. 2002). This phenomenon is involved in the pathogenesis of degenerative tendinopathies such as with achillodynia and degenerative rotator cuff lesions (Lou et al., 1997). The development of hypertrophic, biomechanical inferior, replacement tissue is caused by recurrent microtrauma.

2.4 Influence of growth factors

Cellular growth factors and cytokines play key roles during embryonic tissue differentiation and during wound healing (Gabra et al, 1994; Goomer et al. 2000; Grotendorst et al., 1985; Hudson-Goodman et al., 1990; Mason & Allen 1941). Growth factors are known to stimulate cell differentiation, chemotaxis, angiogenesis, and extracellular cell matrix synthesis (Mason & Allen 1941; Nakamura et al., 1996; Nakamura et al., 1998). Furthermore, these factors regulate cellular synthesis and the secretion activity from matrix components and influence in this manner the course and results of would-healing (Gabra et al., 1994; Lou et al., 1997). The diversity of the cytokinetic characteristics lends credence to the concept that these growth factors are potentially capable of modulating the tendon healing processes, resulting in better healing (Mason & Allen 1941).

The influence of growth factors on tendon healing has been investigated through comparative studies of the profiles of cytokines of injured and normal tendons. It has been shown that wounding and inflammation provoke release of growth factors (Nakamura et al., 1996; Nakamura et al., 1998; Party et al 1978).

2.4.1 PDGF

However, healing tendons have increased PDGF-concentrations (Enzura et al., 1996; Nakamura et al., 1996; Nakamura et al., 1998). Under the influence of PDGF, rates of fibroblasts proliferation, chemotaxis and collagen synthesis are somewhat elevated (O'Brien T, 1992). However, patellar tendon fibroblasts show higher proliferation after the addition of bFGF in vitro (Coombs et al., 1980)

As Molloy wrote at his review, PDGF describes a group of dimeric polypeptide isoforms made up from three types of structurally similar subunits. Its activity is mediated through its interaction with two related tyrosine kinase receptors, one of which binds all three PDGF chains, and the other binds only one (Ronnstrand et al). Work by Duffy et al. (1995) has shown that PDGF is elevated in the healing canine digital flexor tendon, suggesting a role in the healing process. It is thought to play a significant role in the early stages of healing, at which time it induces the synthesis of other growth factors, such as IGF-I (Lynch et al, 1989). In vitro studies by Yoshikawa and Abrahamsson (2001) on PDGF have further demonstrated that this growth factor also plays an important role during tissue remodelling. PDGF was observed to stimulate both collagen and non-collagen protein production, as well as DNA synthesis, in a dose-dependent manner.

One theory that has been put forward as to how PDGF increases protein production involves its induction of TGFβ-1 expression (Pierce et al., 1989). However, in vivo studies by Hildebrand et al. (1998) in which the PDGF isomer PDGF-BB was applied to the healing MCL of the rabbit with and without TGFβ-1 showed no such complementary effect. In fact, addition of PDGF-BB and TGFβ-1 together resulted in poorer healing (as determined by ultimate load, energy absorbed to failure, and ultimate elongation values) than addition of PDGF-BB alone. Stimulation of DNA synthesis by PDGF has also been postulated to occur through a growth factor second messenger. In this case, increases in PDGF have been shown to result in up-regulation of IGF-I and IGF receptors, that once activated stimulate DNA synthesis (Lymch et al 1989). A significant amount of the PDGF produced for this end is thought to come from an exogenous source, probably from platelets (Tsuzaki et al., 2000).

Interestingly, the level of stimulation has been shown to be specific to the site and type of tendon examined. In studies by Yoshikawa and Abrahamsson (2001) DNA synthesis was stimulated to higher levels in intermediate compared with intrasynovial tendons, and protein synthesis was higher in proxi- mal intrasynovial tendon segments than in extrasynovial peroneal tendon segments (Molloy et al, 2003).

2.4.2 VEGF

VEGF is required for the formation of the initial vascular plexus early in granulation tissue development and contributes to vascular bud formation and endotheliocyte migration during neo-vascularization, which occurs at the primary stage of tendon healing. However, his results suggest that VEGF deteriorated tendon properties via vessel formation and destruction of the collagen network while TGF-β enhanced the tendon mechanical properties.

VEGF is not normally found in adult tendon, but is expressed in the healing tendon, alongside with increased expression of the VEGF receptors 1 and 2 in areas with great microvascular density (Petersen et al., 2003b)[18]. When added to a healing tendon, VEGF increases the vascularization from 1 to 8 weeks after rupture (Hou et al., 2009)[7]. Although the mechanical properties are better at 1 week, the difference is no longer significant after only 2 weeks (Zhang et al., 2003)[29]. Since prior to the formation of new vessels there is an increase of matrix metalloproteases and the vascular tissue has inferior mechanical properties compared to a tendon, this may explain the afore mentioned observation. Our findings suggest that VEGF is tightly controlled during at least 8 weeks in tendon healing without big increases or decreases in concentration, but possibly with a slight decrease up to 8 weeks. TGF-β may exert some control over the expression of VEGF by depressing it (Hou et al., 2009)[7], but other pathways such as endostatin are also possible (Pufe et al., 2003)[20].

2.4.3 TGF-β

TGF-β1 is known to play an important role in the healing process of injured tendon by directing the fibroblast migration (Roberts et al.,1988), neovascularization and secretion of extracellular matrix proteins like procollagen type I and III (Kashiwagi et al., 2004).

When TGF is added to the healing tendon, it has been shown to induce the expression of collagen I and III and also improve the mechanical properties of the tendon, seemingly accelerating the healing process (Hou et al., 2009; Kashiwagi et al., 2004). It may be that a single exposure to TGF-β in sufficient dosage is already enough to mobilize and differentiate additional mesenchymal stem cells (Kashiwagi et al., 2004). Normally TGF-β is expressed early in a healing tendon in the process of inflammation and reorganization at 4 and 7 days, whereafter the expression decreases at 2 and 4 weeks (Chan et al., 2003). Loading and mobilization of the tendon seem to decrease the expression of TGF-β (Eliasson et al., 2009), possibly reducing the initial inflammation in the healing tendon. At the end stage of tendon healing TGF-β may also promote the apoptosis of fibrocytes (Jorgensen et al., 2005; Lui et al., 2007). In our one studies we observe a high concentration of TGF-β initially, which then decreased for 2 and 4 weeks and then increase massively at 8 weeks, possibly reflecting the initial inflammation and activation of cells, followed by an intermediary period and then the remodeling of the tendon with increased apoptosis of no longer necessary cells. The results are similar to those for the rat rotatory cuff (Würgler-Hauri et al., 2007), although we observe a steeper increase at 8 weeks.

2.4.4 BMP-12

Several BMPs are able to induce bone and cartilage formation in animals by influencing the differentiation of mesenchymal progenitor cells along the cartilage, or bone lineage (Ducy & Karsenty, 2000; Wozney 1998). However, BMP-12, a human homologue of growth and differentiation factor 7 (GDF-7), does not induce bone or cartilage, BMP-12 induces the formation of tendon and ligament tissue (Enzura et al., 1996; Lou et al., 2001; Wolfman et al., 1997). Therefore, BMP-12 plays an important role in tendon healing. In order to optimize tendon healing it seems to be important to have a high level of expression of collagen type I. Corresponding to this fact there must also be a transition from the initial production of collagen type III to type I.

A natural course of BMP-12 expression has been measured in loaded rat achilles tendons although without the plantaris tendon to act as an internal splint which would mechanically stabilize the healing tendon in the early stages (Eliason et al., 2008). The resulting expression patterns have suggested an initially high expression of BMP-12 at the beginning of tendon healing at 3 days, followed by a decrease at 8 days even below the normal expression and up to 21 days a further slight decrease. At the same time loading of the healing tendon showed a decrease of the expression of follistatin, an inhibitor of BMP-12 (Eliason et al., 2008). Our data accordingly also shows an initially higher concentration of BMP-12 and subsequent decrease after 2 weeks. Because we have measured the concentration directly as opposed to the cellular expression, the time points are somewhat shifted, and it may be that the higher concentration of BMP-12 acts in a negative feedback loop to prevent further BMP-12 expression. The effects of BMP-12 when added in a tendon healing model include the increase of tendon callus and the improvement of mechanical properties such as overall strength and stiffness, both after 1 week (Forslund et al., 2003; Majewski et al., 2008). However BMP-12 added during the first week of healing leads to a more organized tendon tissue (Murray et al., 2007), higher volumes of collagen I and an earlier shift of fibroblasts to fibrocytes (Majewski et al., 2008). Our results thus suggest a tightly controlled BMP-12 concentration, which possibly helps to coordinate the newly produced cells during proliferation in the early healing period. This is also seen with the rat rotatory cuff (Würgler-Hauri et al., 2007), yet we do not see an increase in concentrations after 8 weeks, again possibly reflecting the difference in both tendons.

2.4.5 bFGF

Use of bFGF in a healing tendon has been shown to increase cellularity early in the healing process (Chan et al., 2008). While reducing expression of collagen I and III in the first week (Thomopoulos et al., 2010), it increased both after two weeks (Sahoo et al, 2010), again suggesting a prolonged phase of proliferation, associated with a higher repair potential in a normally bradytrophic tissue. Extracellular matrix changes associated with bFGF are an increase of lubricants and matrix metalloproteases during the first week, supposedly creating the space needed for the additional tenoblasts and tenocytes (Thomopoulos et al., 2010). The initial increase in bFGF we have observed in our study may thus reflect an early phase of the healing process, which provides the tenocytes and fibroblasts needed for the repair of the extracellular matrix by stimulating their proliferation. This is in accordance with the study done in the rat rotatory cuff (Würgler-Hauri et al., 2007), but we have not observed the increase of bFGF after 8 weeks which possibly reflects one of the many differences of the achilles tendon and rotatory cuff.

2.4.6 IGF

During the initial repair process and the inflammatory phase, upregulation of growth factors and cytokines such as insulin-like growth factor-1 (IGF-1) stimulate the migration and proliferation of fibroblasts and inflammatory cells to the wound site (James et al., 2008; Kurtz et al., 1999; Tsuzaki et al., 2010). Several studies have shown that IGF-I is locally increased during and after inflammation following soft tissue injury, both at the mRNA and protein levels, and is associated with a corresponding up-regulation of its receptors (Bos et al., 2001; Edwall et al., 1989; Fortier et al.; 2001; Molloy et al., 2003; Rubini et al., 1994 Sciore et al., 1998; Tsuzaki et al., 2000; Vogt et al., 1998). James mentioned, that Insulin-like growth factor-1 may be stored as an inactive precursor protein in normal tendon and, upon injury, enzymes release the growth factor to exert its biological activity. During the later phases such as remodeling, IGF-1 stimulates synthesis of collagen and other extracellular matrix components; studies in vitro have shown that the effects of IGF-1 on matrix metabolism are dose dependent (James et al., 2008). As Molloy stated, its primary roles seem to be to stimulate the proliferation and migration of fibroblasts and other cells at the site of injury, and to subsequently increase the production of collagens and other extracellular matrix structures in these cells during the remodelling stages. Because IGF-I is such a versatile and widespread signal molecule, it has numerous and varied activities during tendon healing, particularly when working in concert with other growth factors. As with many other cytokines, synergism with other molecules is important for its stimulatory acivity. It is thought that IGF-I works to promote cell proliferation when in the presence of other growth factors, such as the PDGF isomer PDGF-BB (Molloy et al., 2003).

Repair phase	Activity	Growth Factor
Inflammatory	Stimulates recruitment of fibroblasts and	IGF-1
	inflammatory cells to the injury site	TGF-β
	Regulation of cell migration	PDGF
	Expression and attraction of other growth factors (e.g. IGF-1)	VEGF, bFGF
	Angiogenesis	
Proliferative	Cell proliferation (DNA synthesis)	IGF-1, PDGF, TGF-β,
	Stimulates synthesis of collagen and ECM	bFGF, GDF-5,-6,-7
	components	IGF-1, PDGF, bFGF
	Stimulates cell-matrix interactions	TGF-β, bFGF
	Collagen Type III synthesis	TGF-β, GDF-5,-6,-7
Remodelling	ECM remodelling	IGF-1
	Termination of cell proliferation	TGF-β
	Collagen type I synthesis	TGF-β, GDF-5,-6,-7

Table 2. Tendon repair phases with biological characteristics and ensuing molecular events that are regulated by several cytokines or growth factors (from James et al., 2008)

2.4.7 Platelet-rich plasma

Lately platelet-rich plasma is being progressively used to treat musculoskeletal conditions. Within their alpha granules and dense granules platelets have a rich store of factors and cytokines. Among others the alpha granules contain PDGF, TGF-β, IGF-1, VEGF, and EGF, whereas the dense granules contain neuromodulators and inflammatory modulators such as histamine and serotonin. By exposure to collagen, thrombin, or calcium platelets release these growth factors and cytokines (Fufa et al., 2008; Rodeo et al., 2010). For the treatment of chronic Achilles tendinopathy a randomized, double blind, placebo-controlled trial demonstrated no significant differences between patients managed with either platelet-rich plasma or saline solution injections (DeVos et al., 2010; Rodeo et al., 2010). In a prospective, randomized trial platelet-rich-fibrin-augmented rotator cuff repairs showed increased vascularization compared to the control group six but not twelve weeks postoperatively (Rodeo et al., 2010). Repaired superficial digital flexor tendons in front limbs of horses had a higher failure strength and greater elastic modulus 24 weeks postoperatively after being treated with platelet rich plasma compared to the control group with only saline injection. Histologically the platelet-rich plasma group demonstrated better collagen organization and increased metabolic activity (Bosch et al., 2010).

2.4.8 Autologeous conditioned serum

During our own studies on 80 male Sprague Dawley rats we found a marked increase of collagen type I and a decrease of collagen type III in animals treated with ACS (Majewski et al. 2009). An increased content of type III collagen in the fibers would tend to reduce their tensile strength (Jozsa et al, 1984; Jozsa et al, 1990; Maffulli et al, 2000; Matthew & Moore, 1991). ACS-treated animals showed markedly more mature, thick reddish/orange collagen fibers at weeks 2 and 8 postoperatively as compared with controls and quantitative evaluation of collagen type III showed a three fold reduced level of this collagen at weeks 1, 2 and 8. This finding is in agreement with the reports of Aspenberg and Virchenko who documented a beneficial effect of platelet concentrate administration on the histological appearance of the healing tendon, with a concomitant increased tendon callus strength and stiffness by about 30% after week 1, an improvement which persisted for as long as 3 weeks after the injection (Aspenberg & Virchenko, 2004; Wright-Carpenter et al2004). Despite the improved collagen synthesis, which is apparent from the significantly greater tendon thickness at weeks 1, 4 and 8, stiffness was significantly (P=0.038) increased at week 4.

In summary, it is clearly evident that ACS injections accelerate the rate of organization of repair tendon tissue. ACS injections apparently do not critically limit inflammatory signals of the early healing phase but supplement critical growth factors that are present in serum in limiting concentrations. The biologically active components in ACS are responsible for the observed accelerated Achilles tendon healing (Majewski et al. 2009).

2.5 Natural course of healing

The normal course of tendon healing with an emphasis on growth factor expression has been studied for various models of tendon pathology, including rotatory cuff tears and Achilles tendon ruptures in a rat model as well as in tenocyte cultures. However only a few studies have focused on the expression of several growth factors over time. Indications as to which growth factors are at work at what time during tendon healing can be emerge from studies on the temporal growth factors expression during unaided healing as well as from studies on the effects of local growth factor administration. As to the unaided healing, Würgler-Hauri and coworkers documented the temporal expression of growth factors in tendon-to-bone healing in a rat supraspinatus model using immunohistochemical staining . Their results show that all growth factors measured increase at weeks 1 and 2, as well as at week 8 (Würgler-Hauri et al., 2007).

As tendons vary greatly in function and structure, we studied the expression during healing over time of bFGF, BMP-12, VEGF and TGF-β in a rat Achilles tendon healing model. After surgically introduced, immunohistological analysis was performed for 1, 2, 4 and 8 weeks of healing. Results showed a high initial concentration of bFGF and BMP-12, which sank rapidly after 2 weeks, while VEGF remained elevated just slowly decreasing over time and TGF-β even increased after 8 weeks. The observed difference compared to the rotatory cuff model is maybe due to tendon-to-tendon versus tendon-to-bone healing.

3. Tissue engineering

3.1 Cytokines modulation

Growth factors and cytokines modulate the differentiation of tendons during embryogenesis and play also an important role during the healing process of tendons (Grotendorst, 1988; Hudson-Goodman et al, 1990). In healthy canine flexor tendons an increased expression of bFGF was measured whereas the amount of PDGF was increased in healing tendons (Duffy et al, 1995). Under the influence of PDGF an increased chemotaxis of fibroblasts, proliferation rate and collagen synthesis was observed (Grotendorst, 1988; Pierce et al, 1995). bFGF caused an increased fibroblast proliferation in in vitro Achilles tendons and an angiogenic effect of bFGF has been shown (Chan, et al; 1997; Gabra et al, 1994). During tendon embryogenesis bone morphogenetic proteins (BMP), especially BMP 12 and 13 cause the expression of elastin and collagen I. In animal studies BMP 12 induced healing of the patellar tendon (Möller et al, 2000). In in vitro studies an increased mRNA expression of type I collagen by the transforming growth factor * family (TGF*) has been shown.

3.2 Scaffolds

Lately biocompatible and biodegradable scaffolds are also used in tissue engineering of tendon healing. They are thought to mimic native extracellular matrix in the beginning of tendon healing. Moreover scaffolds are supposed to hold cells that are involved in the tendon healing either by being implanted or chemo-attracted to the scaffold (Gott et al, 2011). Combination of scaffolds and tenocytes led to superior histologic and biomechanical repairs in flexor tendons compared to scaffolds without tenocytes. However, the use of scaffolds might impair tendon gliding within narrow synovial sheaths (Adams et al., 2006; Cao et al., 2002; Gott et al, 2011). The positive affect of scaffolds in Achilles tendon and rotator cuff repair is rather achieved by combination with other tissue engineering modalities e.g. growth factors or bio-adhesiv coat than by the structural support alone, which showed to be not sufficient enough. Pericardium or dermal tissue that was augmented with a bioadhesive coating showed improved biomechanical properties compered to control in an Achilles tendon model (Brodie et al., 2011; Derwin et al., 2006; Gott et al, 2011). In a rabbit model a polyglycolic-acid scaffold combined with fibrin was seeded with Achilles tenocytes and then implanted in a defined Achilles tendon defect. Compared to the control groups (scaffold alone and without scaffold) macroscopic and microscopic appearance was superior. Unfortunately no biomechanical testing was performed in this study (Stoll et al. 2011). In massive rotator cuff tear a functioning scaffold model is desirable. Nevertheless the goal remains to create a tension-free, anatomical repair that restores the footprint as scaffolds have not yet shown to have the adequate biomechanical power (Nho et al, 2010). In this field more research is need to be done. Rather the biologic part than the mechanic part seems to be promising in the use of scaffolds.

3.3 Gene intervention

Several investigators have studied gene transfer to tendons. Three model systems have been used; the patellar tendon of the knee (Gerich et al., 1996; Nakamura et al., 1996), the digital flexor tendon (Goomer et al. 2000, Lou et al., 1996, Lou et al., 1997, Lou et al., 2001), and the Achilles tendon (Dai et al., 2003). In these model systems, repair strength and gap formation of the tendon scar is important while with digital flexor tendons a second, equally important issue is adhesion formation between the healing tendon and the surrounding tendon pulley sheaths.

The investigators considered the feasibility of gene transfer in digital flexor tendons of chickens and dogs, and patellar or Achilles tendons of rats [5,13,25,35]. Nakamura, used the

HVJ-liposome construct to deliver ß-galactosidase to a rat patellar tendon [35]. Approximately 7% of the cells were ß-galactosidase positive 7 days after injection and this decreased to 0.2% of cells 56 days after injection. [35]. Digital flexor tendons in dogs and chickens were modified using cationic liposomes and expression vector containing ß-galactosidase to enhance transfection [13,25]. 6 days later the transfection efficiencies were reported as 100% [13]. The authors reported no evidence of immune response.

The second digital flexor tendon model was that of chicken flexor tendons [25]. ß-galactosidase expression was detected in the tendon and tendon sheath at 3, 30 and 75 days after injection. An estimated 2-5% of cells were ß-galactosidase positive and most of these cells were on the surfaces of the tendon and tendon sheath [25]. The fourth study used a transected rat Achilles tendon model without suturing to evaluate ß-galactosidase expression [5]. At 4 days after transection, recombinant adenovirus carrying LacZ was placed in the transection site. The authors detected ß-galactosidase expression up to 17 days after injection and 21 days after transection. Transduction rates increased with higher doses of injected virus [5]. The previous four studies with tendons used direct injection of the vectors in or around the tendons.

Oezkan investigated the feasibility of intra-arterial injection of HVJ-liposomes for transfecting cells of the patellar tendon and found that between 8 and 12% of the cells positive [38].

Three studies have tried to manipulate the healing environment of tendons [27,26,36]. Two studies evaluated digital flexor tendons, studying adhesion formation and the tendon scar strength [26,27]. Lou, used gene intervention to manipulate the healing environment of chicken digital flexor tendons to investigate tendon adhesions [26].

Lou did a study in chicken digital flexor tendon. They used an adenoviral construct with BMP-12 to transduce primary chicken tendon cells in vitro. Collagen Type I synthesis was increased 30% by cells transduced with the adenoviral-BMP-12 construct when compared to control cells or cells transduced with an adenovirus-ß-galactosidase construct. While there were no significant differences in the ultimate failure force or the stiffness at 2 weeks, by 4 weeks these values for adenoviral-BMP-12 group were approximately significant greater than the values of adenoviral- ß-galactosidase group [27].

4. How to best improve tendon healing with growth factors

Tendon ruptures and tears are slow healing common injuries that are often treated surgically with unsatisfactory results for some patients. As the biology of the healing process and how it is influenced by growth factors become clear, one can consider introducing biological therapy into clinical use. As data on the effect of specific recombinant growth factors were mainly obtained from studies in different animal models of tendon healing, these are difficult to compare.

In our own studies we have compared the benefits of three different approaches of tendon healing influenced by growth factors: TGF-β as an example for multifunctional growth factors inducing a wide range of cellular responses, BMP-12 as example for the specific induction of tendon and ligament tissue, and a growth factor cytokine mix derived from serum and activated platelets as an example for biological therapy.

We hypothesized that the interplay of numerous growth factors and cytokines contributes to optimal tendon healing. We reasoned that the growth factors normally present in serum and released by activated platelets could approximate the growth factor/cytokine mix seen by the injured tendon better then when single growth factors are applied.

The transected rat Achilles tendon was used for the evaluation of the effect of all growth factors. Doing a pre-study, staining intensity for BMP-12, bFGF, TGF β, and VEGF showed that all these factors are highly expressed at the early stage of healing.

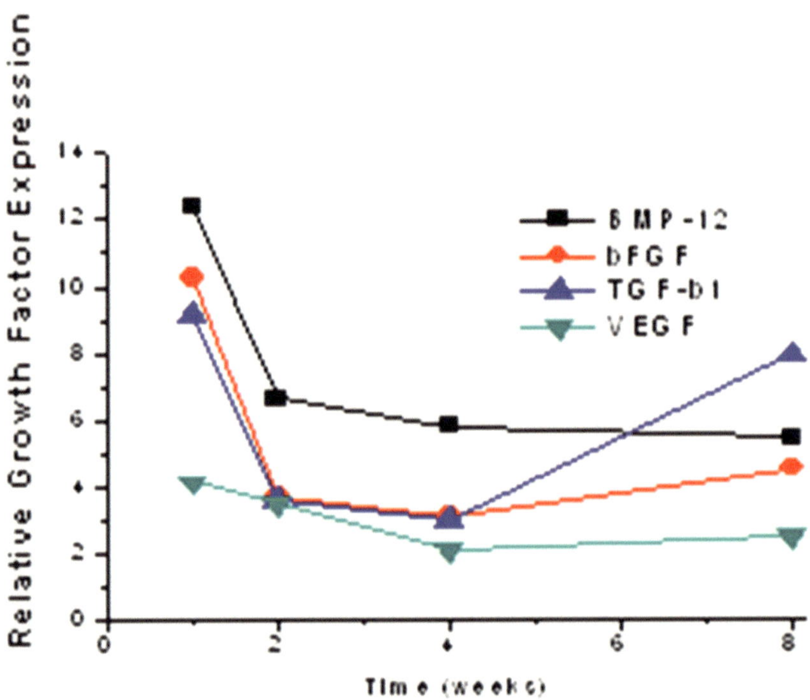

Fig. 1. Relative Growth factor Expression in correlation to the time after injury. A relative high expression was measured within the first week. TGF-β tends to rise again after 4 weeks, whereas the others remain at a stable level after two weeks.

Therefore, BMP-12 cDNA, and separately TGF-β cDNA were introduced at the time of surgery and activated serum (ACS) was injected at the time of tendon surgery as well as 24 and 48 postoperatively. Animals were sacrificed 1, 2, 4, and 8 weeks later and Achilles tendon tendon-bone units were collected. Biomechanical testing, histochemical and immunochemical analyses of regenerate sections were performed using standard techniques.

4.1 Biomechanical testing

TGF-β: Biomechanical testing of the healing rat Achilles tendon showed an increased maximum load. The maximum failure load was significantly increased one week after surgery, compared to the control (p=0.0012), and was also somewhat higher after 4 and 8 weeks. Tendon stiffness was significantly higher after one week.

BMP-12: Tendons exposed to BMP-12 showed significantly greater strength (P=0.0379) than controls at 1 week. Tendon stiffness was significantly higher at 1, 2 and 4 weeks Control tendons, in contrast, only achieved normal stiffness values after 8 weeks.

AS: AS-tendons reached stiffness values 4 weeks earlier than the controls. There were no differences in maximum load to failure between groups up to week 8.

4.2 Histology

TGF-β: Histological examination showed a much more organized and homogeneous pattern of collagen fibers over all time points compared to controls. The fibers grew to bigger bundles much earlier with a higher degree of collagen crimp.

BMP-12: The Histological examination was quite similar compared to TGF-β group. However, after 8 weeks, there was one tendon with an enchondral ossification at the experimental group.

AS: Collagen fibers were apparent as early as week 1 postoperatively. These collagen fibers were visibly thicker and more bundled than in all other tendon at this stage. The trend toward better organized collagen continued in week 2 and 4. At 8 weeks postoperatively, the tendons had a smooth appearance resembling very much normal tendons with small fibrocartilaginous areas in the center of the stress areas.

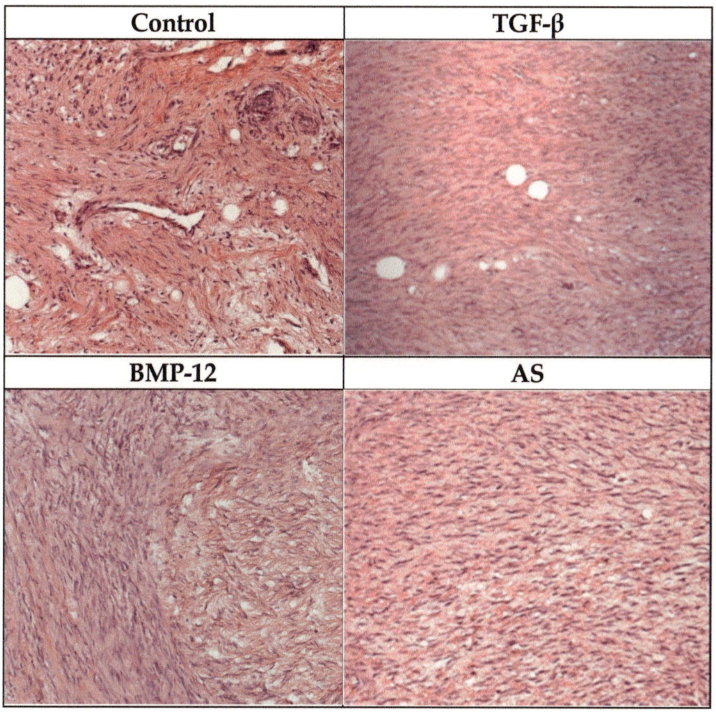

Fig. 2. Effect of different Growth Factor on the histologic appearance of the repair site. Sections were made from tendons recovered 1 week after surgery and stained with hematoxylin and eosine. Magnification: x200.

4.3 Collagen

Control tendons contain mainly collagen I, and approximately 3% collagen III. In regenerates formed under the influence of TGF-β this collagen ratio is reached after 2 weeks. With BMP-12 stimulation a collagen III content of 3% is reached by week 4, and with AS by week 8.

	Biomechanics	Ratio collagen type I/III	Histology
TGF-β	+	+++	+
BMP-12	++	++	+/(-)
Biological therapy (ACS)	-	+	+++

Table 3. Effects of growth-factors on transected rat Achilles tendon healing

4.4 Conclusions

Our data indicate that the mix of growth factors and cytokines in activated serum yields superior tendon healing than single growth factors as judged by histological appearance of the regenerate. However, growth factors BMP-12 and TGF-β yielded better biomechanical results and more favorable collagen expression ratios, respectively. As tendon ruptures and tears are slow healing injuries, the quality of life and economic productivity of patients is often diminished for weeks. It would benefit patients greatly if the healing process could be accelerated and improved by biological intervention as appears possible from our data. At present it is not clear which of the approaches of growth factor delivery is most promising as each of them yields better outcomes in a respect or another (collagen ratio, histological appearance, biomechanical properties). Further studies are needed to determine whether it is possible to obtain normal tendon tissue by growth factor application.

5. Abbreviations

ACS	autologous conditioned serum
bFGF	basic fibroblast growth factor
BMP	bone morphogenetic protein
CDMP	cartilage-derived morphogenetic protein
EGF	epidermal growth factor
GDF	growth and differentiation factor
IGF	insulin-like growth factor
PDGF	platelet-derived growth factor
PRP	platelet-rich plasma
TGF-β	transforming growth factor beta
VEGF	vascular endothelial growth factor

6. References

Adams JE, Zobitz ME, Reach JS, Jr, An KN, Steinmann SP. Rotator cuff repair using an acellular dermal matrix graft: an in vivo study in a canine model. Arthroscopy 22:700-709, 2006.

Aspenberg P, Virchenko O. Platelet concentrate injection improves Achilles tendon repair in rats. Acta Orthop Scand 2004;75:93-99

Birk, O.E., & Trelstad R.L. (1984). Extracellular compartments in matrix morphogenesis: Collagen fibril, bundle and lamellar formation by corneal fibroblasts. J Cell Biol, Vol. 99, No. 6 (December 1984), 2024-2033, ISSN: 0021-9533

Bos PK, van Osch G, Frenz DA, et al. Growth factor expression in cartilage wound healing: temporal and spatial immunolocal- ization in a rabbit auricular cartilage wound model. Osteoarthritis Cartilage 2001; 9 (4): 382-9

Bosch G, van Schie HT, de Groot MW, Cadby JA, van de Lest CH, Barneveld A, van Weeren PR. Effects of platelet-rich plasma on the quality of repair of mechanically induced core lesions in equine superficial digital flexor tendons: A placebo-controlled experimental study. J Orthop Res 2010, Feb;28(2):211-7

Cao Y, Liu Y, Liu W, Shan Q, Buonocore SD, Cui L. Bridging tendon defects using autologous tenocyte engineered tendon in a hen model. Plast Reconstr Surg 110:1280-1289, 2002

Chan BP. Chan KM, Mafulli N (1997) Effect of basic fibroblast growth factor: an in vitra study of tendon healing. Clin Orthop 342: 239-247

Chan KM, Fu SC, Wong YP, Hui WC, Cheuk YC,and Wong MW.Expression of transforming growth factor beta isoforms and their roles in tendon healing. Wound Repair Regen, 16(3):399–407, May-Jun 2008

Coombs RHR, Klenerman L. Narcisi p. Nichols A, Pope FM (1980) Collagen typing in Achilles tendon rupture. J Bone Joint Surg Br 62: 258

Dai Q, Manfield L, Wang Y, Murrell GAC (2003) Adenovirus-mediated gene transfer to healing tendon – enhanced efficiency using a gelantin sponge. J Orthop Res 21: 604-609

Derwin KA, Baker AR, Spragg RK, Leigh DR, Iannotti JP. Commercial extracellular matrix scaffolds for rotator cuff tendon repair. Biomechanical, biochemical, and cellular properties. J Bone Joint Surg 88:2665-2672, 2006

De Vos RJ, Weir A, van Schie HT, Bierma-Zeinstra SM, Verhaar JA, Weinans H, Tol JL. Platelet-rich plasma injection for chronic Achilles tendinopathy: a randomized controlled trial. JAMA. 2010; 303:144-9

Ducy P, Karsenty G. (2000) The family of bone morphogenetic proteins. Kidney Int. 57:2207-2214

Duffy FJ, Seiler JG, Gelberman RH, Hergrueter CA. Growth factors and canine flexor tendon healing: Initial studies in uninjured and repair models. J Hand Surg Am 1995, Jul;20(4):645-9

Edwall D, Schalling M, Jennische E, et al. Induction of insulin- like growth factor I messenger ribonucleic acid during regener- ation of rat skeletal muscle. Endocrinology 1989; 124: 820-5

Eliasson P, Fahlgren A, and Aspenberg P. Mechanical load and bmp signaling during tendon repair: a role for follistatin? Clin Orthop Relat Res, 466(7):1592– 1597, Jul 2008

Eliasson P, Andersson T, and Aspenberg P. Rat achilles tendon healing: mechanical loading and gene expression. J Appl Physiol, 107(2):399–407, Aug 2009

Enzura Y, Rosen V, Nifuji A (1996) Introduction of hypertrophy in healing patellar tendon by implantation of human recombinant BMP 12. J Bone Min Res 11: 401

Forslund C, Rueger D, and Aspenberg P. A comparative dose-response study of cartilage-derived morphogenetic protein (cdmp)-1, -2 and -3 for tendon healing in rats. J Orthop Res, 21(4):617–621, Jul 2003.

Fortier LA, Balkman C, Sandell LJ, et al. Insulin-like growth factor-I gene expression patterns during spontaneous repair of acute articular cartilage injury. J Orthop Res 2001; 19 (4): 720-8

Fufa D, Shealy B, Jacobson M, Kevy S, Murray MM. Activation of platelet-rich plasma using soluble type I collagen. J Oral Maxillofac Surg. 2008; 66:684-90

Gabra N, Khiat A, Calabres (1994) Detection of elevated basic fibroblast growth lactat during early hours of in vitra angiogenesis using a fast ElISA immunoassay. Biochem Biophys Res Commun 205:1423-1430

Gerich TG, Kang R, Fu FH, Robbins PD, Evans CH (1996) Gene transfer to rabbit patellar tendon: potential for genetic enhancement of tendon and ligament healing. Gene Ther 3: 1089-1093

Goomer RS, Maris TM, Gelberman R, Boyer M, Silvia M, Amiel D (2000) Nonviral in vivo gene therapy for tissue engenieering of articular cartilage and tendon repair. Clin Orthop Relat Res. 379 Suppl: 189-200

Gott M, Ast M, Lane LB, Schwartz JA, Catanzano A, Razzano P, Grande DA. Tendon phenotype should dictate tissue engineering modality in tendon repair: a review. Discov Med. 2011 Jul;12(62):75-84

Grotendorst GR, Martin GR, Pencer D (1985) Stimulation of granulation tissue forma- tion by PDGF in normal and diabetic rats. J Clin Invest 76: 2323-2329

Grotendorst GR (1988) Growth factors as regulators of wound repair. Int Tissue React 10: 337-344

Hefti F, Stoll TM. (1995) Healing of ligaments and tendons. Orthopade. 24:237-45

Hildebrand KA, Woo SL, Smith DW, et al. The effects of platelet-derived growth factor-BB on healing of the rabbit medial collateral ligament: an in vivo study. Am J Sports Med 1998; 26 (4): 549-54

Hou Y, Mao Z, Wei X, Lin L, Chen L, Wang H, Fu X, Zhang J,and Yu C.Effects of transforming growth factor-beta1 and vascular endothelial growth factor 165 gene transfer on achilles tendon healing. Matrix Biol, 28(6):324–335, Jul 2009.

Hudson-Goodman P, Girard N, Jones MB (1990) Wound repair and the potential use of growth factors. Heart Lung 19: 379-384

James, R., Kesturu, G., Balian, G. & Chhabra, A.B. Tendon: biology, biomechanics, repair, growth factors, and evolving treatment options. J Hand Surg Am 33, 102-12 (2008)

Janqueira LC, Bignolas G, Brentani RR (1978) Picrosirus staining plus polarization microscopy, a specific method for collagen detection in tissue sections. Histochemical Journal 11: 447-455

Jorgensen HG, McLellan SD, Crossan JF, and Curtis AS. Neutralisation of tgf beta or binding of vla-4 to fibronectin prevents rat tendon adhesion following transection. Cytokine, 30(4):195–202, May 2005.

Jozsa L, Kannus P, Reffy A, Demel Z (1984) Fine structural alterations of collagen bets in degenerative tendinopathy. Arch Orthop Trauma Surg 103: 47-51

Jozsa L, Reffy A, Kannus P, Demel S, Elek E. Pathological alterations in human tendons. Arch Orthop Trauma Surg 1990;110:15-21

Kashiwagi K, Mochizuki Y, Yasunaga Y, Ishida O, Deie M, and Ochi M. Effects of transforming growth factor-beta 1 on the early stages of healing of the achilles tendon in a rat model. Scand J Plast Reconstr Surg Hand Surg, 38(4):193–197, 2004.

Kurtz CA, Loebig TG, Anderson DD, DeMeo PJ, Campbell PG. Insulin-like growth factor I accelerates functional recovery from Achilles tendon injury in a rat model. Am J Sports Med 1999;27:363–369.

Laemmli UK (1970) Cleavage of structural proteins during assembly of the head of bacteriophage T4. Nature 227:680-685

Lou J, Manske PR, Aoki M, Joyce ME (1996) Adenovirus-mediated gene transfer into tendon and tendon sheath. J Orthop Res 14: 513-517

Lou J, Kubota H, Hotokezaka S, Ludwig FJ, Manske PR (1997) In vivo gene transfer and overexpression of focal adheasion kinase (pp125FAK) mediated by recombinant adenovirus-induced tendon adheasion formation and epitenon cell change. J Orthop Res 15: 911-918

Lou J, Tu Y, Burns M, Silva MJ, Manske P: BMP-12 gene transfer augmentation of lacerated tendon repair. J Orthop Res 19:1199-1202, 2001

Lui PP, Cheuk YC, Hung LK, Fu SC, and Chan KM. Increased apoptosis at the late stage of tendon healing. Wound Repair Regen, 15(5):702–707, Sep-Oct 2007.

Lynch SE, Colvin R, Antoniades HN. Growth factors in wound healing: single and synergistic effects on partial thickness porcine skin wounds. J Clin Invest 1989; 84 (2): 640-6

Maffulli N, Ewen SW, Waterston SW, et al. (2000) Tenocytes from ruptured and tendinopathic achilles tendons produce greater quantities of type III collagen than tenocytes from normal achilles tendons. An in vitro model of human tendon healing. Am J Sports Med: 499–505

Maffulli N, Moller HD, Evans CH (2002) Tendon healing: can it be optimised? Br J Sports Med 36:315-316

Majewski M, Betz O, Ochsner PE, Liu F, Porter RM, and Evans CH. Ex vivo adenoviral transfer of bone morphogenetic protein 12 (bmp-12) cdna improves achilles tendon healing in a rat model. Gene Ther, 15(16):1139–1146, Aug 2008.

Majewski M, Ochsner PE, Liu F, Flückiger R, Evans CH. Accelerated healing of the rat Achilles tendon in response to autologous conditioned serum. Am J Sports Med. 2009 Nov;37(11):2117-25.

Mason ML, Allen HS (1941) The rate of healing of tendons: an experimental study of tensile strength. Ann Surg 113: 424-459

Matthew CA, Moore MJ. Regeneration of rat extensor digitorum longus tendon: the effect of a sequential partial tenotomy on collagen fibril formation. Matrix 1991;11:259-268

Möller HD, Evans CD, Robins PD, Fu FH (1998) Gene therapy in orthopaedic sports medizine. In: Chan KM, Fu FH, Kurosaka M, Mafulli N, Rolf C, Liu 5 (eds) Controversies in ortho- paedic sports medicine. Williams-Wilkins, Hong Kong, pp 577-588

Möller HD, Evans CH, Maffulli N. Aktuelle aspekte der sehnenheilung. Der Orthopäde 2000;29(3):182-7

Molloy, T.; Wang Y., & Murrell, G. (2003). The roles of growth factors in tendon and ligament healing. Sports Med, Vol 33:381-394.

Murray DH, Kubiak EN, Jazrawi LM, Araghi A, Kummer F, Loebenberg MI, and Zuckerman JD. The effect of cartilage-derived morphogenetic protein 2 on initial healing of a rotator cuff defect in a rat model. J Shoulder Elbow Surg, 16(2):251–254, Mar-Apr 2007

Nakamura N, Horibe S, Matsumoto N, Tomita T, Natsuume T, Kaneda Y, Shino K, Ochi T (1996) Transient introduction of a foreign gene info healing rat patellar ligament. J Clin Invest 97: 226-231

Nakamura N, Shino K, Natsuume T, Horibe S, Matsumoto N, Kaneda Y, Ochi T (1998) Early biological effect of in vivo gene transfer of platelet-derived growth factor (PDGF)-B into healing patellar ligament. Gene Therapy 5:1165–1170

Nho SJ, Delos D, Yadav H, Pensak M, Romeo AA, Warren RF, MacGillivray JD. Biomechanical and biologic augmentation for the treatment of massive rotator cuff tears.Am J Sports Med. 2010 Mar;38(3):619-29. Epub 2009 Sep 23.

O'Brien T (1992) Functional anatomy and physiology of tendons. Clin Sports Med 11: 505-520

Özkan I, Shino K, Nakamura N , Natsuume T, Matsumoto N, Horibe S, Tomita T, Kaneda Y, Ochi T (1999) Direct in vivo gene transfer to healing rat patellar tendon by intra-arterial delivery of haemaggglutinating virus of Japan Liposomes. Trans Orthop Res Soc 29: 63-67

Party DAD, Barnes GRG, Craig AS (1978) A comparison of the size distribution of collagen fibrils in connective tissues as a function of age and a possible relationship between fibril size distribution and mechanical properties. Proc Roy Soc London 203: 305-321

Petersen W, Pufe T, Zantop T, Tillmann B, Mentlein R. (2003) Hypoxia and PDGF have a synergistic effect that increases the expression of the angiogenetic peptide vascular endothelial growth factor in Achilles tendon fibroblasts. Arch Orthop Trauma Surg.123: 485-488

Petersen W, Pufe T, Unterhauser F, Zantop T, Mentlein T, and Weiler A. The splice variants 120 and 164 of the angiogenic peptide vascular endothelial cell growth factor (vegf) are expressed during achilles tendon healing. Arch Orthop Trauma Surg, 123(9):475–480, Nov 2003

Petersen W, Varoga D, Zantop T, Hassenpflug J, Mentlein R, Pufe T. (2004) Cyclic strain influences the expression of the vascular endothelial growth factor (VEGF) and the hypoxia inducible factor 1 alpha (HIF-1alpha) in tendon fibroblasts. J Orthop Res. 22:847-853

Pierce GF, Mustoe T, Lingelbach J, et al. Platelet-derived growth factor and transforming growth factor-beta enhance tissue repair activities by unique mechanisms. J Cell Biol 1989; 109 (1): 429-40

Pierce GF, Tarpley JE, Tseng J (1995) Detection of platelet-derived growth factor (PDGF)- IW in actively healing human wounds treated with recombinant PDGF-pp and absence of PDGF in chronic nonhealing wounds. J Clin Invest 96: 1336-1350

Pufe T, Petersen W, Kurz B, Tsokos M, Tillmann B, and Mentlein R. Mechan- ical factors influence the expression of endostatin–an inhibitor of angiogenesis–in tendons. J Orthop Res, 21(4):610–616, Jul 2003.

Rodeo SA, Delos D, Weber A, Ju X, Cunningham ME, Fortier L, Maher S. What's New in Orthopaedic Research. J Bone Joint Surg Am. 2010; 92:2491-2501

Roberts AB, Flanders KC, Kondaiah P, Thompson NL, Obberghen-Schilling E, Wakefield L, Rossi P, de Crombrugghe B, Heine U, Sporn MB: Transforming growth factor beta: biochemistry and roles in embryogenesis, tissue repair and remodeling, and carcinogenesis. Recent Prog Horm Res 44:157-197, 1988

Ronnstrand L, Heldin C. Mechanisms of platelet-derived growth factor-induced chemotaxis. Int J Cancer 2001; 91 (6): 757-62

Rubini M, Werner H, Gandini E, et al. Platelet-derived growth factor increases the activity of the promoter of the insulin-like growth factor-I (IGFI) receptor gene. Exp Cell Res 1994; 211: 374-9

Sahoo S, Toh SL, and Goh JC. A bfgf-releasing silk/plga-based biohybrid scaffold for ligament/tendon tissue engineering using mesenchymal progenitor cells. Biomaterials, 31(11):2990–2998, Apr 2010.

Sciore P, Boykiw R, Hart DA. Semi-quantitive reverse trans- criptase polymerase chain reaction analysis of mRNA for growth factors and growth factor receptors from normal and healing rabbit medial collateral ligament tissue. J Orthop Res 1998; 16: 429-37

Stoll C, John T, Conrad C, Lohan A, Hondke S, Ertel W, Kaps C, Endres M, Sittinger M, Ringe J, Schulze-Tanzil G. Healing parameters in a rabbit partial tendon defect following tenocyte/biomaterial implantation. Biomaterials. 2011 Jul;32(21):4806-15. Epub 2011 Apr 6.

Tsuzaki M, Brigman BE, Yamamoto J, Lawrence WT, Simmons JG, Mohapatra NK, et al. Insulin-like growth factor-I is expressed by avian flexor tendon cells. J Orthop Res 2000;18:546–556.

Thomopoulos S, Das R, Sakiyama-Elbert S, Silva MJ, Charlton N, and Gelberman RH. bfgf and pdgf-bb for tendon repair: controlled release and biologic activity by tendon fibroblasts in vitro. Ann Biomed Eng, 38(2):225–234, Feb 2010.

Tsuzaki M, Brigman B, Yamamoto J, et al. Insulin-like growth factor-I is expressed by avian flexor tendon cells. J Orthop Res 2000; 18 (4): 546-56

Vogt PM, Lehnhardt M, Wagner D, et al. Growth factors and insulin-like growth factor binding proteins in acute wound fluid. Growth Horm IGF Res 1998; 8 Suppl B: 107-9

Wolfman NM, Hattersley G, Cox K, Celeste AJ, Nelson R, Yamaji N, Dube JL, DiBlasio-Smith E, Nove J, Song JJ, Wozney JM, Rosen V: Ectopic induction of tendon and ligament in rats by growth and differentiation factors 5, 6, and 7, members of the TGF-beta gene family. J Clin Invest 100:321-330, 1997

Wozney JM, Rosen V: Bone morphogenetic protein and bone morphogenetic protein gene family in bone formation and repair. Clin Orthop Relat Res26-37, 1998

Wright-Carpenter T, Opolon P, Appell HJ, Meijer H, Wehling P, Mir LM. Treatment of muscle injuries by local administration of autologous conditioned serum: animal experiments using a muscle contusion model. Int J Sports Med 2004;25:582-587

Würgler-Hauri CC, Dourte LM, Baradet TC, Williams GR, and Soslowsky LJ. Temporal expression of 8 growth factors in tendon-to-bone healing in a rat supraspinatus model. J Shoulder Elbow Surg, 16(5 Suppl):198–203, Sep-Oct 2007

Yoshikawa Y, Abrahamsson S. Dose-related cellular effects of platelet-derived growth factor-BB differ in various types of rabbit tendons in vitro. Acta Orthop Scand 2001; 72 (3): 287-92

Zhang F, Liu H, Stile F, Lei M P, Pang Y, Oswald T M, Beck J, Dorsett-Martin W, and Lineaweaver W C. Effect of vascular endothelial growth factor on rat achilles tendon healing. Plast Reconstr Surg, 112(6):1613–1619, Nov 2003.

4

Noninsertional Achilles Tendinopathy – Treatment with Platelet Rich Plasma (PRP)

Marta Tarczyńska and Krzysztof Gawęda
NZOZ Arthros, Nałęczów
Orthopaedic Surgery and Traumatology Department,
Medical University of Lublin
Poland

1. Introduction

1.1 Tendinopathy pathology

Various forms of overload pathology of the Achilles tendon constitutes the usual source of pain within the posterior surface of the peripheral part of the calf, occurring without particular traumatic cause.

This condition affects patients across ages groups *(1,2)*. Both the location of the pathological lesions and their nature are different from each other *(3)*. Pain is usually reported approximately 2 - 6 cm above the junction of the tendon and calcaneal tubercle. This condition has been called **noninsertional tendinopathy** *(4)*.

As opposed to the above, the pathological processes that develop at the Achilles tendon attachment site on the calcaneus have been called **insertional tendinopathy**, and are less frequent. Initially, both conditions were jointly referred to as **Achilles tendinitis,** supposedly to explain the inflammatory origin of lesions in the calcaneal tendon and its insertion point.

According to Schepsis this was an incorrect approach, resulting from insufficient knowledge and understanding of the variable nature of pathological lesions in the course of these processes *(5)*. **Clinical, imaging or histological features of inflammation were rarely observed** *(6,7)*. **These were only seen in the peritendineum** *(7)*. **They were often symptomless, did not cause any complaints and were only found by accident** *(5)*. However, considering the results of other studies, lesions in the Achilles tendon were found to involve neurogenic inflammation *(8,9)*.

The usual cause of pain is related to an increase in the number of cells in the tendon, and an increase of their activity, thus resulting in an increased volume of extracellular substance. The collagen fibre pattern and neovascularisation process are thus corrupted *(10)*. **There is no evidence indicating the development of prostaglandin-mediated inflammation.** Sometimes, fatty degeneration or mucin deposits are observed in the Achilles tendon *(5)*.

Such incomplete knowledge of the aetiopathogenesis has led to many misunderstandings regarding nomenclature, and even treatment methods *(5,11)*. **The term tendinitis,**

indicating an inflammatory aetiology, is therefore correct only for the neurogenic origin that is not a frequent feature of the pathomorphological picture. It has been replaced in the literature by terms such as tendinosis or tendinopathy, used interchangeably *(5)*.

1.2 Tendinopathy aetiology

Tendinopathy may develop as a result of a single cause, or result from the overlapping effects of multiple causative factors. These always lead to an overload of the Achilles tendon. It is believed that a sudden, short-term increase of loads may be one of the causes of the developing lesions. In a similar manner, an overload may also result from an increased duration or frequency of physical training loads.

As a result of an increased frequency of training sessions, the rest intervals become shorter, thus reducing the chances for regeneration and self-repair of any micro-injuries that may have occurred.

An undoubted increase of the risk of Achilles tendinopathy occurs when the training shoes are replaced with new, often uncomfortable or even improper ones that force a pronation position of the foot. Subjecting the foot to loads in forced tarsal overpronation causes an increase of the forces transmitted through the calcaneal tendon.

Own observations in ultrasonography studies show that lesions usually occur within the section of the calcaneal tendon formed by the medial head of the gastrocnemius muscle. Running on a hard and uneven surface forces substantial and suddenly changing tensions within the Achilles tendon that lead to the formation of lesions within its internal structure.

Seasonal changes of the surface on which the patient walks or trains on an everyday basis also play an important role. Excessively tense or weakened muscles of the calf, subjected to regular loads, also sometimes cause the development of calcaneal tendon overload lesions.

A limited range of motion in the ankle joint is a similar risk factor. Inappropriate motor training methods, especially insufficient muscular warm-up prior to training, improper stretching of calf muscles or their abrupt cooling after effort increase the risk of Achilles tendinopathy.

1.3 Tendinopathy symptoms

1.3.1 Clinical

Patients' complaints and physical symptoms of noninsertional Achilles tendinopathy are variable, depending on the severity and extent of the lesions. It has also been found that the duration of the pathological processes has an impact on the severity and features of the complaints.

The most frequent and unspecific symptom is moderate to severe pain in the area of the calcaneal tendon, located proximally from its attachment to the calcaneus. The painful section of the tendon usually shows evidence of a nodule- or spindle-like thickening.

The thickened areas are very painful at palpation. Pressure sensitivity can be increased following a period of rest, especially at night. Patients report stiffness of the ankle joint during its first movements. A reduction of strength and range of plantar flexion of the foot is observed. A sensations of heaviness of the affected limb is a common complaint.

Considering the pain incidence and intensity, noninsertional Achilles tendinopathy is classified into 4 stages. Stage I features pain that occurs only following effort, especially running. Patients with stage II report pain both before and after running. Complaints slightly decrease while running. Stage III includes pain during any activity, significantly reducing the duration and levels of achievable loads. In stage IV, pain occurs during normal everyday activity that increases the pain intensity or extends its duration.

1.3.2 Imaging

Standard radiological imaging are not useful in supporting the diagnostics and imaging of tendinopathy lesions of the calcaneal tendon. Only imaging techniques that are capable of showing the differences in soft tissue structure may be helpful in diagnosing and monitoring the course of tendinopathy of the Achilles tendon.

Ultrasonography (US) and magnetic resonance imaging (MRI) are the golden standard in tendinopathy imaging. Due to its availability, ultrasonography is the most frequently used method. Various ultrasonography options and variants are useful.

The most frequent ultrasonographic symptoms of tendinopathy are focal thickening of the tendon, hypoechogenic intratendinous foci and evidence of rupture of the fibrillar structure of tendons. A thickening of the peritendon and tendon sliding restriction during active movements of the foot are less frequent. Ultrasonography with the Power Doppler (PDUS) and Color Doppler (CDUS) options usually shows no substantial abnormalities while clinical symptoms last. Healing symptoms are clearly visible in the form of increased number of vascular pulses within the tendon, and in the immediate vicinity of the tendon *(12)*. Fig. 1, 2.

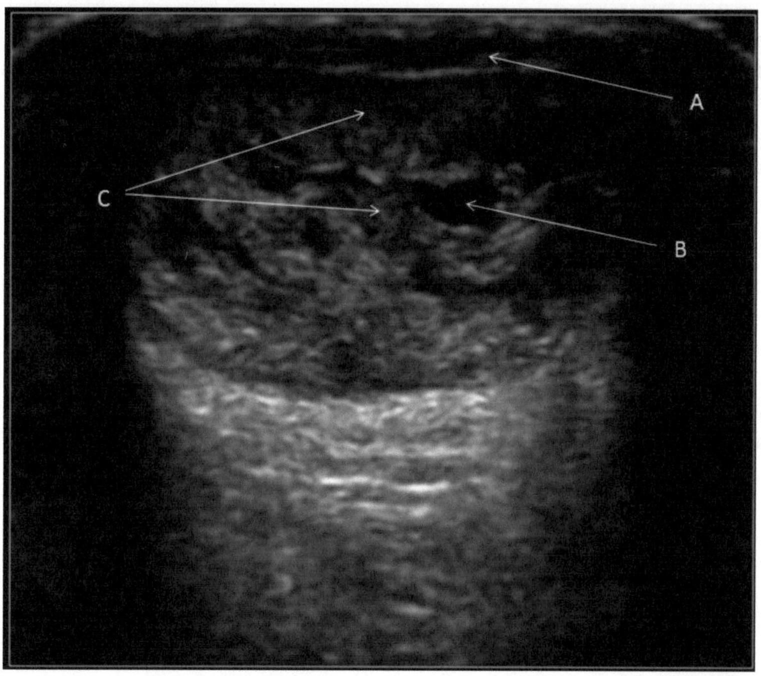

Fig. 1. Transverse US view of Achilles tendinopathy: A - peritendon thickening, B - area of fibrillar rupture, C - hypoechogenic foci.

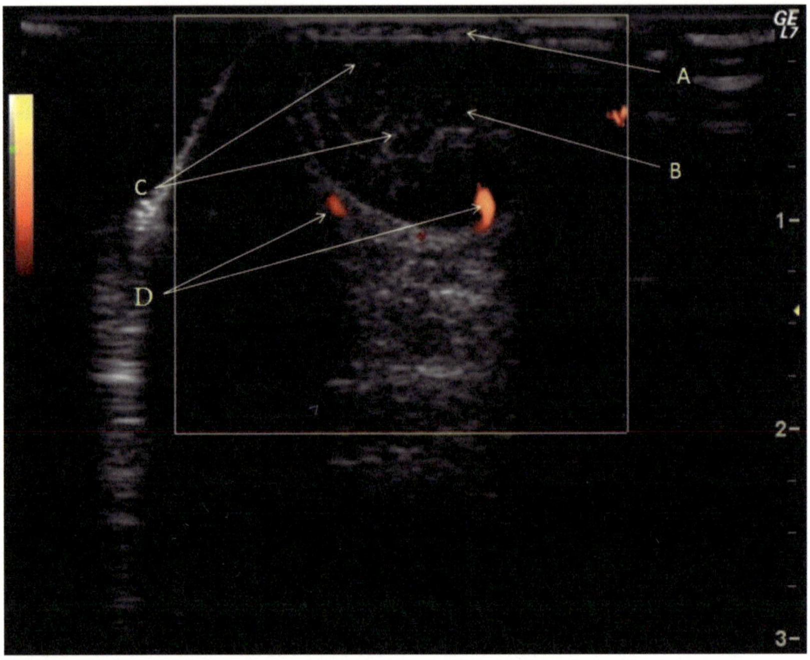

Fig. 2. Transverse PDUS view of Achilles tendinopathy: A - peritendon thickening, B - area of fibrillar rupture, C - hypoechogenic foci, D - vascular pulses.

Comparing with US studies, MRI scans are more sensitive in differentiating adjacent healthy and affected tissues. MRI scans allow the imaging of a selected area in various planes and a more detailed evaluation of the internal structure of the investigated organ. Its costs and limited availability make MRI scans useful only for the evaluation of cases that are doubtful in terms of diagnostics, or following various invasive treatments that may blur the ultrasonographic image *(13)*.

1.4 Treatment methods

Many authors stress the necessity to properly match the management method with the cause of tendinopathy, its severity and previously used therapies *(14,15)*. Conservative management should be used for initial stages of progression of the disease, and mainly in the younger patients. The need to resort to surgery increases with the duration of the complaints, their intensity and the age of the patient *(16,17)*. A complete management algorithm depending on the above mentioned criteria has been presented by Alfredson *(18)*.

The management principle for every Achilles tendon tendinopathy is to discontinue previous motor activity at the origin of tendinopathy lesions, and resting of the patient.

Initial management should include stretching and eccentric training exercises. Appropriate footwear with heel elevation should be used, and the easiest way to achieve this is to insert a cork wedge into one's own shoe. With pain complaints resolved, the programme of returning to training should be modified. If such management proves ineffective, unloading with elbow crutches becomes necessary.

At the same time, various forms of physiotherapy are used, such as ultrasounds, magnetic fields, laser or ultrasonic shock wave *(19)*. Some centres sometimes recommend massage and immobilisation in carefully selected orthoses. Cast immobilisation is rarely used.

In the event of a failure of the physiotherapy management methods, many patients undergo steroid injections into the affected areas in the vicinity of the calcaneal tendon. The alleviation of complaints reported following such management is temporary. As the nature of the lesions within the tendon has usually no inflammatory origin, it is difficult to expect the improvement to be long-lasting, as it only translates into reduced pain.

It is also sometimes recommended to proceed with injections of products causing obliteration of the vessels formed in the neovascularisation processes that are seen in the course of tendinopathy.

The inefficacy of subsequent treatment modalities, especially in middle and older age patients, leads to the performance of various surgical interventions. The value of surgical management is generally positively perceived by the patients, especially in subjects who had previously been treated without effect using other management methods *(20,21)*.

We have implemented a different management method at our Centre. It consists in a local administration of autologous leukocyte- and platelet-rich plasma (L-PRP) under direct ultrasonographic imaging control into evidenced lesions within the calcaneal tendons *(22)*.

2. Objective

The objective of this paper is to evaluate the efficacy of noninsertional Achilles tendinopathy treatment using local injections of autologous leukocyte- and platelet-rich plasma.

3. Material

Evaluation involved the treatment of 29 patients aged 24 through 53 years, 42 years on average. Patients included 11 women and 18 men. In 5 subjects, lesions involved bilateral calcaneal tendons. Therefore, 34 tendons were subjected to this treatment. Sport or motor activities exceeding the average loading level for a given age group were seen in 7 subjects. Metabolic abnormalities in the form of diabetes were noted in one patient.

The period of complaints preceding treatment with autologous leukocyte- and platelet-rich plasma ranged from 5 to 21 months, on average 14 months. L-PRP injections were used following failure of other forms of treatment in all subjects. Initially, immobilisation was used in 11 patients, and all subjects underwent various physiotherapy procedures. One-time steroid injections were given in 9 cases. The above patient characteristics indicate that some patients underwent various therapies at subsequent phases of the course of the disease. None of the previously used therapies proved effective in eliminating the tendinopathy symptoms. There were no periods of substantial reduction of complaints. The follow-up period for patients treated with L-PRP until their last follow-up visit exceeded 1 year in all subjects.

4. Method

Evaluation involved randomly selected patients among those reporting for treatment at the outpatient clinic of the hospital, presenting with pain of the posterior surface of calf circumference. Based on an initial interview and physical examination, subjects with clinical features of noninsertional tendinopathy were selected. The main inclusion criteria were symptoms lasting time longer than 5 months and fail of previously employed non-invasive treatment modalities. Patients with insertional tendinopathy symptoms and those without previous courses of physiotherapy, rest, heel elevation and limb unload were excluded from the study and referred to these treatment forms.

All patients presented painful thickening of the Achilles tendon, at a level at least 2 cm above its insertion point into the calcaneal tubercle. There was evidence of painful restriction of plantar and dorsal flexion movements. Conserved ankle pronation and supination movements also caused pain in the peripheral section of the Achilles tendon. An objective functional evaluation was performed using the AOFAS scale for the posterior section of the foot, and using VISA-A score *(23,24)*.

All the selected patients had radiograms of the ankle joint performed that also included the distal ½ of the calf, using standard radiographic projections. If radiograms were not showing lesions within the skeletal system, ultrasonographic evaluation was performed within the painful area of the calcaneal tendon, using a linear probe with frequencies of 12-15 MHz. Continuity of the entire tendon and its internal structure were verified using ultrasonography. The evaluation focused on seeking out focal continuity ruptures of the fibrillar tendon structure, determining the filling of empty inter-fibrillar spaces, and confirming the presence or absence of tendon oedema and its sheath. The freedom of tendon movement was assessed in a dynamic study. The intensity of vascular flow was evaluated using Power-Doppler within the tendon, its sheath and in its direct vicinity, including the para-insertional area on the calcaneal tubercle and the Kager's triangle.

Peripheral blood morphology and biochemistry tests were performed in subjects to exclude generalised inflammatory symptoms. Fulfilment of all diagnostic criteria allowed the patient to be included in the therapeutic group, upon receipt of the patient's informed consent.

Peripheral blood was taken from subjects selected for treatment, and a thrombocyte preparation was prepared according to the recommendations of the separator manufacturer. The suspension thus obtained was injected under ultrasonographic control into hypoechogenic foci within the area of affected tendon. Fig. 3, 4.

For 3 days following the injection, subjects were recommended to unload the limb, use elbow crutches, and elevate the limb. Within the next 2 weeks, patients used walking sticks, walking with partial loading of the anterior section of the foot, performed passive motor exercises of the ankle joint. During the following 2 weeks, the loading of the foot was gradually increased with concomitant elevation of the heel in the subject's own footwear, with continued passive and active exercises with limb unloading. At 6 weeks following the injection, patients started full loading of the limb without walking sticks. Heel elevation was maintained.

6 weeks after injection, all patients underwent another evaluation of the foot performance based on the AOFAS criteria and with the VISA-A performance scales. A follow-up ultrasonographic evaluation was also performed at that time. The same features were evaluated as during the baseline evaluation. Normal daily activity was recommended if fibrillar regeneration symptoms were seen. Periodic heel elevation was still maintained. Patients were advised against motor activity, even at recreational levels.

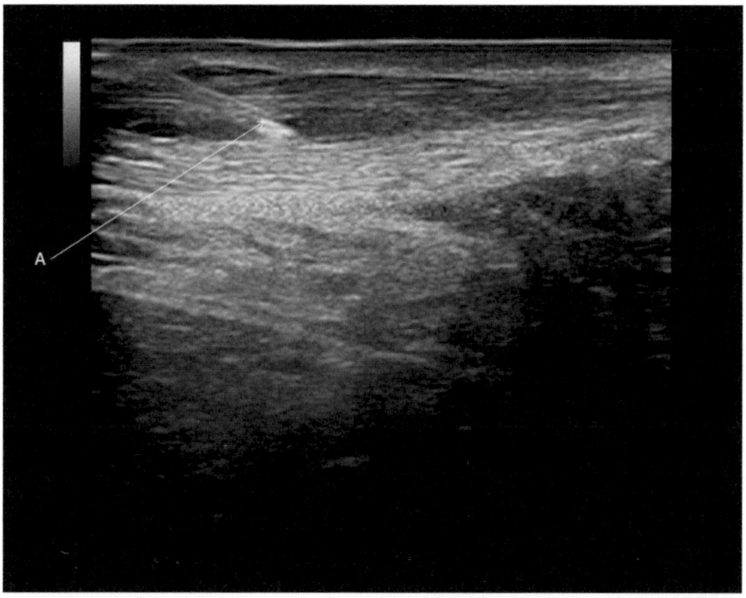

Fig. 3. US longitudinal view demonstrating the needle insertion into the tendon: A - needle.

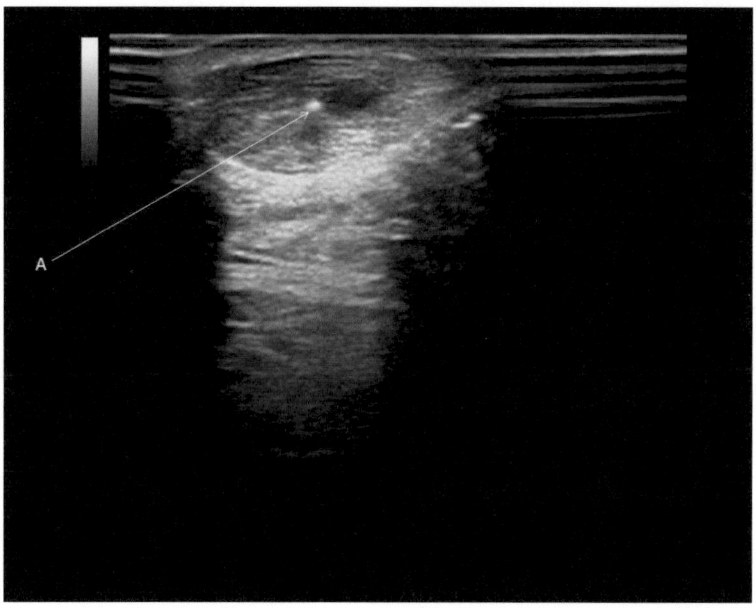

Fig. 4. US transverse view demonstrating the needle insertion into the tendon: A - needle.

Injections were repeated in patients with limited progression of healing reactions seen at ultrasonography evaluations. In the case of 15 treated patients it proved necessary to repeat the injections. Subject who did not require repeat administrations of the preparation between 6 and 12 weeks after the procedure returned to their normal activities, as conducted prior to the onset of the symptoms. Patients who received repeat injections underwent rehabilitation in the same manner as following the first injection.

Subsequent clinical evaluations using functional performance scales and ultrasonographic examinations were conducted in all treated patients 6 and 12 weeks after treatment, as well as 6 and 12 months after treatment. Follow-up continuity is ensured through follow-up visits scheduled once a year.

5. Results

Before starting the therapy, the values for functional assessment using the AOFAS scale for the posterior section of the foot ranged from 28 to 69 points, with 47 points on average. Using the VISA-A scale, patients achieved scores ranging from 6 to 34, with an average of 21 points. Ultrasonographic evaluations in all subjects showed spindle-like thickening of the tendon, also involving the peritendon in 17 cases. Numerous intratendinous ruptures were seen in 8 patients. Isolated fibrillar rupture lesions were observed in 14 other subjects. All evaluated subjects showed hypoechogenic areas within these lesions, 7 of them showed only small hypoechogenic foci. 5 subjects presented a significant restriction of tendon mobility at dynamic evaluation. Four subjects had evidence of foci with significantly reduced echogenicity, potentially consistent with intratendinous hyalinisation. These were patients who had previously received steroid injections into the affected area. There were no patients with inflammatory reaction within the Achilles bursa. Studies with the Power Doppler option showed no evidence of an increased blood supply within the lesions area.

After 6 weeks, AOFAS scores ranged from 64 to 84 points, with an average of 76. VISA-A scores were in the range between 27 and 58 points, 44 on average. Ultrasonographic evaluation in 21 patients showed persistent thickening of the tendon at the location of intratendinous ruptures. The thickness of the peritendon remained increased in 14 subjects. In most patients a discreet reduction of the size of hypoechogenic foci was seen. No alteration of the tendon movement range was seen in 3 patients. In 23 subjects, a substantial increase of the number of vascular flow signals was seen, as compared with baseline.

Evaluations at 12 weeks showed AOFAS scores in the range between 68 and 100 points, 90 on average, and VISA-A scores ranging from 48 to 98, with an average of 87 points. Regression of the spindle-like tendon thickening was seen in ultrasonographic evaluations, observed in 11 subjects. In 6 subjects, a decreased thickness of the peritendon was noted, as compared to the evaluation at 6 weeks. In 13 subjects, the areas of fibrillar continuity rupture faded out. In 11 subjects, small hypoechogenic areas were seen, reduced in size as compared with previous evaluations. Four tendons showed evidence of residual presence of fibrillar rupture areas. Power Doppler evaluation showed an increased number of vessels within the tendinopathy area.

After 6 months, AOFAS scores ranged from 72 to 100 points, with an average of 91. VISA-A scores ranged from 64 to 100 points, with an average of 90 points. 25 subjects were freed from local pain and thickening of the Achilles tendon. These tendons showed reduced thickness at ultrasonographic evaluation. A reduction of the peritendon thickness was also noted. Its previous abnormal thickening was only seen in 3 subjects. These subjects also had isolated intratendinous hypoechogenic foci. Two subjects still showed discreet evidence of rupture of the tendon fibres. All treated patients showed normal, symmetrical mobility of the Achilles tendon. The number of vascular signals within the tendon itself was reduced, but remained unchanged within the vicinity of the tendon, as compared with the previous evaluation.

After a year, AOFAS scores ranged from 80 to 100 points, with an average of 94 points. Patients achieved VISA-A scores in the range of 78-100 points, and an average of 93 points. Ultrasonographic evaluations showed thickening of the tendons in 3 subjects. Peritendon thickening also persisted in 3 subjects. There were no intratendinous fibrillar ruptures, however small, focal reduced echogenicity areas were still seen in 3 evaluations. PDUS studies showed a further decrease of the number of vascular signals within the tendons and their vicinity.

Further annual evaluations for up to 4 years showed neither a recurrence of the complaints nor a deterioration of clinical assessment scores in any of the evaluated patients. All treated patients achieved pain resolution and full motor function in everyday activities. Periodic pain following sports was seen in 7 patients, however at reduced levels, as compared with the pretreatment period.

6. Discussion

Eccentric exercises recommended by Woodley and Fahlstrom did not lead to a cure in our patients in their management prior to L-PRP injections *(25,26)*. Based on a review of 697 bibliographic items, Rompe assessed the value of NSAIDs administration, steroid injections, heel supports and various forms of physical therapy in the treatment of Achilles tendinopathy *(27)*. He concluded that their efficacy is similar to that of the placebo effect, while the results are comparable to those achieved in groups of subjects receiving no treatment at all.

Surgical management methods proposed by Schepsis have not been verified in our material, as we have not used surgical management *(5)*. Similarly, we are unable to evaluate the efficacy of endoscopic management proposed by Steenstra *(28)*.

Treatment of chronic tendinopathy of the calcaneal tendon using L-PRP injections provided alleviation or withdrawal of disease symptoms in all our patients. Observations made by other authors are thus confirmed; other authors noticed an improvement of tendon repair capacities following local administration of growth factors.

Kurtz reported anti-inflammatory effects of IGF-1 in the healing of sectioned tendons, while Sanchez reported a similar effect following the application of PRGF *(29,30)*. Anitua reported in studies conducted in sheep that blood platelet concentrates administered onto fibrin matrices accelerate and shape the proliferation of active tendon cells and stimulate neovascularisation *(31)*.

Schnabel et al. have shown in experimental studies on a model of equine tendons that an increased concentration of blood platelets and growth factors they release causes an increased expression of genes responsible for tendon repair *(32)*. Mishra presented promising experiences in the treatment of tendinopathy of wrist and hand extensor tendon insertion points in the area of the lateral epicondyle of humerus using buffered platelet-rich plasma *(33)*.

On the other hand, the observation made in Power Doppler ultrasonographic evaluations is puzzling. Baseline evaluations have shown no differences in the number of vascular flow signals as compared to the healthy side. In subsequent follow-up evaluations after 6 and 12 weeks, the number of vascular flow signals gradually increased, and the process did not stop in evaluations performed after 24 weeks within tissues surrounding the tendons. However, at that time, the number of vascular impulses within the tendons themselves was significantly inferior. Knoblach reports that micro-circulation anomalies may be a cause for developing tendinopathy *(34)*. He considers that extra-capillary venous hyperaemia is one feature of this process, without impact, however, on the tissue oxygenation levels.

Resolving clinical symptoms, increasing tendon thickness at rupture sites, and a decreased thickening of the tendon and peritendon, with fading out of hypoechogenic foci, as observed in ultrasonography evaluations, show substantial repair efficacy following local injection of autologous thrombocyte gel into the affected area of calcaneal tendon. The lack of appropriate number of the randomised controls is the week point of the study. Good and very good results after L-PRP injections were gained in the group of patients with affected Achilles tendons who had previously employed heel elevation, rest, limb unloading or physiotherapy and didn't improved. In this term, the role of these treatment modalities in the course post L-PRP injections presumably is small and were advised for pain and mechanical protection or patient's comfort soon after needle manipulation around the heal. The statistically significant increase in functional assessment scores, with simultaneous complete absence of complications, show the high therapeutic value of this method.

7. Conclusions

1. In author's opinion local administration of autologous platelet-rich plasma in chronic noninsertional tendinopathy of the Achilles tendon provides substantial reduction and in most cases a complete withdrawal of the disease symptoms.
2. The treatment results of noninsertional Achilles tendinopathy with direct L-PRP injection into affected area are higher then other non-invasive treatment modalities.
3. Positive early and medium term treatment results require further follow-up and well controlled, randomised studies.

8. References

[1] Mahieu NN, Witvrouw E, Stevens V et al. *Intrinsic Risk Factors for the Development of Achilles Tendon Overuse Injury: A Prospective Study.* Am J Sports Med. 2006; 34:226-35

[2] Clement DB, Taunton JE, Smart GW, McNicol KL. *A survey of overuse running injuries.* Physician Sportsmed. 1981; 9:47-58

[3] Astrom M, Rausing A. *Chronic achilles tendinopathy: a survey of surgical and histopathic findings.* Clin Orthop Rel Res. 1995; 316:151-64

[4] Puddu G, Ippolito E, Postucchini F. *Classification of Achilles Tendon Disease.* Am J Sports Med. 1976; 4:145-50

[5] Schepsis AA, Jones H, Haas AL. *Achilles Tendon Disorders in Athletes.* Am J Sports Med. 2002; 30:287-305

[6] Clancy WG Jr. *Tendon Trauma and Overuse Injuries in Sports-Induced Inflamation: Clinical and Basic Science Concepts.* Chicago, AAOS, 1989

[7] Leach RE, Jones S, Wasilewski S. *Achilles Tedinitis.* Am J Sports Med. 1981; 9:93-8

[8] Hart DA, Frank CB, Bray RC. *Inflammatory processes in repetitive motion and overuse syndromes: potential role of neurogenic mechanisms in tendons and ligaments.* In: Gordon SL, Blair SJ, Fine LJ, eds. Repetitive motion disorders of the upper extremity. Rosemont, IL: American Academy of Orthopaedic Surgeons. 1995, 247-62

[9] Scott A, Khan KM, Cook JL et al. *What do we mean by the term "inflammation"? A contemporary basic science update for sports medicine.* Br J Sports Med. 2004; 38:372-80

[10] Alfredson H, Thorsen K, Lorentzon R. *In situ microdialysis in tendon tissue: high levels of glutamate, but not protoglandin E2 in chronic Achilles tendon pain.* Knee Surg Sports Traumatol Arthrosc. 1999; 7:378-81

[11] Fox JM, Blazina ME, Jobe FW et al. *Degeneration and rupture of the Achilles Tendon.* Clin Orthop. 1975; 107:221-4

[12] Gawęda K, Tarczyńska M, Krzyżanowski W. *Treatment of Achilles Tendinopathy with Platelet-Rich Plasma.* Int J Sports Med. 2010; 31:577-83

[13] Shalabi A, Kristoffersen-Wilberg M, Svensson L et al. *Eccentric Training of the Gastrocnemius-Soleus Complex in Chronic Achilles Tendinopathy Results in Decreased Tendon Volume and Intratendinous Signal as Evaluated by MRI.* Am J Sports Med. 2004; 32:1285-96

[14] Kannus P. *Tendon pathology: basic science and clinical applications.* Sports Exerc Inj. 1997; 3:62-75

[15] Kader D, Saxena A, Movin T et al. *Achilles tendinopathy: some aspects of basic science and clinical management.* Br J Sports Med. 2002; 36:239-49

[16] Paavola M, Kannus P, Paakkala T et al. *Long-term prognosis of patients with Achilles tendinopathy. An observational 8-year follow-up study.* Am J Sports Med. 2000; 28:634-42

[17] Kvist M. *Achilles tendon injuries in athletes.* Sports Med. 1994; 18:173-201

[18] Alfredson H, Cook J. *A treatment algorithm for managing Achilles tendinopathy: new treatment options.* Br J Sports Med. 2007; 41:211-6

[19] Luscombe KL, Sharma P, Maffulli N. *Achilles Tendinopathy.* Trauma. 2003; 5:215-25

[20] Vulpiani MC, Guzzini M, Ferretti A. *Operative Treatment of Chronic Achilles Tendinopathy.* Int Orthop. 2003; 27:307-10

[21] Maffulli N, Testa V, Capasso G et al. *Results of Percutaneous Longitudinal Tenotomy for Achilles Tendinopathy in Middle- and Long-distance Runners.* Am J Sports Med. 1997; 25:835-40

[22] Ehrenfest DM, Rasmusson L, Albrektsson T. *Classification of platelet concentrates: from pure platelet-rich plasma (P-PRP) to leucocyte- and platelet-rich fibrin (L-PRF).* Trends Biotechnol. 2009 Mar; 27(3):158-67

[23] Kitaoka HB, Alexander JJ, Adelaar RS et al. *Clinical Rating System for the Ankle-Hindfoot, Midfoot, Hallux and Lesser Toes.* Foot and Ankle International. 1994; 15:7

[24] Robinson JM, Cook JL, Purdam C et al. *The VISA-A Questionnaire: A valid and reliabile index of the clinical severity of Achilles tendinopathy.* Br J Sports Med. 2001; 35:335-41

[25] Woodley BL, Newsham-West RJ, Baxter GD et al. *Chronic Tendinopathy: Effectiveness of Eccentric Exercise.* Br J Sports Med. 2007; 41:188-98

[26] Fahlstrom M, Jonsson P, Lorentzon R, Alfredson H. *Chronic Achilles Tendon Treated with Eccentric Calf-Muscle Training.* Knee Surg Sports Traumatol Arthrosc. 2003; 11:327-33

[27] Rompe JD, Nafe B, Furia JP, Maffulli N. *Eccentric Loading, Shock-Wave Treatment or a Wait-and-See Policy for Tendinopathy of the Main Body of Tendon Achilles: A Randomized Controlled Trial.* Am J Sports Med. 2007; 35:374-83

[28] Steenstra E, van Dijk CN. *Achilles Tendoscopy.* Foot Ankle Clin. 2006; 11:429-38

[29] Kurtz CA, Loebig TG, Anderson DD et al. *Insulin-Like Growth Fator I Accelerates Functional Recovery from Achilles Tendon Injury in a Rat Model.* Am J Sports Med. 1999; 27:363-9

[30] Sanchez M, Anitua E, Azofra J et al. *Comparison of Surgical Repaired Achilles Tendon Tears Using Platelet-Rich Fibrin Matrices.* Am J Sports Med. 2007; 35:245-51

[31] Anitua E, Sanchez M, Zalduendo M et al. *Autologous Fibrin Matrices: a Potential Source of Biological Mediators that Modulate Tendon Cell Activities.* J Biomed Mater Res A. 2006; 77:285-93

[32] Schnabel LV, Mohammed HO, Miller BJ et al. *Platelet Rich Plasma (PRP) Enhances Anabolic Gene Expression Patterns in Flexor Digitorum Superficialis Tendons.* J Orthop Res. 2007; 25:230-40

[33] Mishra A, Pavelko T. *Treatment of Chronic Elbow Tendinosis With Buffered Platelet-Rich Plasma.* Am J Sports Med. 2006; 10:1-5

[34] Knoblach K, Kraemer R, Lichtenberg A et al. *Achilles Tendon and Paratendon Microcirculation in Midportion and Insertional Tendinopathy in Athletes.* Am J Sports Med. 2006; 34:92-7.

5

Current Strategy in the Treatment of Achilles Tendinopathy

Justin Paoloni
Premier Orthopaedics and Sports Medicine,
University of NSW, Kogarah, Sydney
Australia

1. Introduction

Achilles tendinopathy is a common condition that has a relatively high morbidity in both the general population and in athletes. The most commonly used and accepted theory is that it is a degenerative tendinopathy caused by relative overuse in weightbearing activities, and this is especially the case in chronic cases. In the early stages of symptoms it is more likely that there will be no obvious degenerative changes and this has been termed tendinosis and is considered reversible. Achilles tendinopathy can be a difficult condition to treat, especially when it is chronic, and it is important to address causative factors in the management of this condition to ensure symptom reduction and minimize the risk of recurrence. In order to do this, a sound knowledge of anatomy and pathophysiology is required to accurately assess the musculoskeletal regions impacting on the loading of the Achilles tendon. As with all tendinopathies, the basic principles of evidence based exercise rehabilitation should be the mainstay of treatment. All other therapies should be used as adjuncts to this. Many medications can be trialed as therapy is more recalcitrant cases, but caution must be used to weigh the known risks and benefits and "first do no harm" ("primum nil nocere"). Achilles tendinopathy is a condition that can be frustrating to treat and requires careful management and patience to ensure optimal outcomes.

2. Anatomy

The Achilles tendon is a large strong tendon that joins the calf muscle to the posterior aspect of the calcaneus. The gastrocnemius muscle is formed from two heads that arise from the posterior femur above the knee joint and join in the calf with the soleus muscle, which arises from the posterior tibia and fibula below the knee joint. These two muscles merge to form the Achilles tendon in the mid-calf. The gastrocnemius and soleus muscles and their tendoAchilles are the primary ankle plantarflexors. The soleus component of the Achilles tendon twists medially as its approaches the Achilles insertion and, occasionally, an accessory soleus muscle is present and inserts onto the posteromedial calcaneus separate to the Achilles tendon.

At the insertion onto the posterior calcaneus there are two bursae associated with the Achilles tendon, the retrocalcaneal bursa that slides in the angle between the posterosuperior calcaneal border and the anterior aspect of the distal Achilles tendon (Figure 1), and the retroAchilles bursa that slides between the posterior Achilles tendon at its insertion and the overlying skin and subcutaneous tissue. These bursae have a lubricating function to reduce friction during ankle movement, but can become involved in the pathologic process.

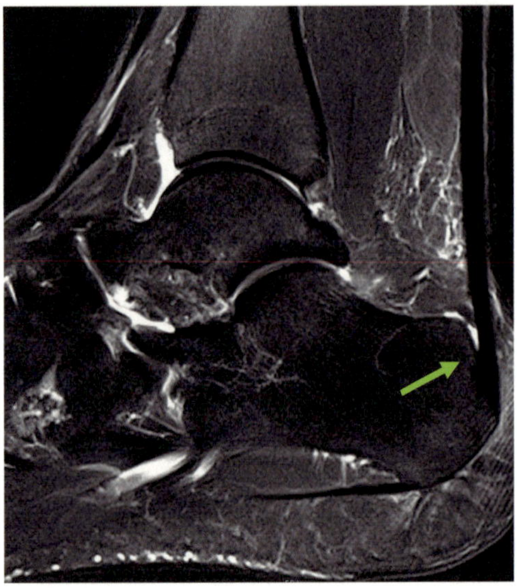

Fig. 1. MRI sagittal image demonstrating the Achilles tendon anatomy. The arrow indicates the Achilles tendon (black) inserting onto the posterosuperior calcaneus and also shows a small fluid collection in the retrocalcaneal bursa (white) between the anterior aspect of the Achilles tendon and the posterosuperior calcaneus.

The Achilles tendon is surrounded by a fine sheath, the paratenon, that is not a synovial sheath but has lubrication and friction reduced properties. It is recognized that the paratenon may be involved in the pathologic process of Achilles tendinopathy, and may contribute to loss of friction reduction and potentially increased tendon fibre strain and thus degeneration.

3. Pathophysiology

Tendons are relatively slow metabolically, with approximately 10-13% of the oxygen uptake of muscle. Tendons heal at a slower rate than muscle and take approximately 100 days (over 3 months) to form biomechanically strong collagenous scar tissue with enough tensile strength and elasticity to accept the forces applied to the Achilles tendon during heavy weightbearing activity such as running or jumping. This slow metabolic rate and slow healing rate have implications for treatment of the Achilles tendon in order to prevent injury recurrence.

Chronic Achilles tendinopathy is almost exclusively a degenerative tendinopathy with histopathologic features of collagen fibre disruption and disorientation (fibre tearing), mucoid degeneration, new blood vessel formation (neovascularisation), and an absence of inflammatory cells. It is due to the absence of inflammatory cells histopathologically that the general descriptor "tendinopathy" is now preferred to the inflammatory descriptor "tendonitis". It should, however, be recognized that the histopathologic description above applies to chronic tendinopathy and it is possible, some may say highly likely, that is the acute stages of Achilles tendon injury there is an inflammatory component in the paratenon and possibly the tendon itself. There may also be symptoms with pathologic changes, this is termed "tendinosis", and is considered a reversible condition due to the lack of observed tendon changes.

Achilles tendinopathy is classified into two types, insertion Achilles tendinopathy that is commonly associated with bursitis, and non-insertional Achilles tendinopathy that is classically location in the relatively hypovascular "watershed" region of the tendon 4-6 cms from the calcaneal insertion. Non-insertional Achilles tendinopathy is rarely associated with bursitis but may have more of an element of paratenon involvement. Recent research has suggested a genetic association between the COL1A1 gene locus and the development of non-insertional Achilles tendinopathy in Caucasian populations in South Africa and in Australia. Other suggested risk factors for the development of Achilles tendinopathy include both intrinsic and extrinsic factors (Table 1). Many of these risk factors and their cause and effect relationship with Achilles tendinopathy remain to be scientifically tested and proven.

Intrinsic Risk Factors	Extrinsic Risk Factors
Genetics (COL1A1) Biomechanical abnormalities: leg length discrepancy subtalar hyperpronation muscle asymmetry/ tightness joint asymmetry/ stiffness joint instability (e.g. lateral ankle laxity, peroneal subluxation) Rheumatic disease: rheumatoid arthritis psoriatic arthritis Collagen disorders Metabolic disorders	Training Insufficient warm-up/ stretching training frequency training intensity training duration training volume monotony of training cross-training Surfaces slopes/ hills/ cambered surfaces change to hard or soft surface unstable surface (e.g. soft sand) Equipment footwear rackets in rackets sports Nutrition Inadequate carbohydrates/ protein Inadequate hydration during exercise Medications: - flouroquinolones (e.g. ciprofloxacin) - anabolic steroids

Table 1. Suggested intrinsic and extrinsic risk factors for Achilles tendinopathy.

It may be that a combination of intrinsic risk factors such as muscle or joint asymmetry of subtalar hyperpronation, when combined with relative overuse of the tendon through repetitive loading and microtrauma, lead to the development of Achilles tendinopathy. Of course, in general, it is difficult to alter intrinsic risks and the major treatment modalities focus of alteration and correction of extrinsic risk factors. History and examination are critical in elucidating intrinsic and extrinsic risk factors and these factors should be corrected, wherever possible, to assist in alleviating symptoms and preventing injury recurrence.

Differential Diagnosis of Posterior Ankle/ Heel Pain
Bony Fracture: os trigonum calcaneal stress fracture Severe's disease (adolescent patients) Joint Tarsal coalition Soft-tissue Impingement syndromes posterior ankle impingement tarsal tunnel syndrome entrapment medial calcaneal nerves sural nerve entrapment Musculotendinous injury peroneal tendon tear/ tenosynovitis / subluxation/ dislocation tibialis posterior tendon tear/ tenosynovitis accessory soleus muscle (Figure 2) Other Referred pain from the lumbar spine Rheumatic disease, especially rheumatoid arthritis or psoriatic arthropathy Metabolic disease (gout, familial hypercholesterolemia)

Table 2. The differential diagnoses of patients presenting with posterior heel pain or ankle pain.

4. Clinical features of achilles tendinopathy

Thorough history and examination is the cornerstone of diagnosis in medicine, and this must be the first step in assessing the Achilles tendon. This is to ensure that the correct diagnosis is made and that risk factors are addressed in the management program to optimize treatment outcomes.

4.1 History

Achilles tendinopathy is relatively common in weightbearing athletes with rates between 5-20% reported in runners. It is a common injury presentation in runners, track and field athletes, and all football players. The classic presentation of Achilles tendinopathy is the insidious onset of posterior heel or calf pain over a few months. There may be pain, swelling, and impairment of function. It may have a relapsing and remitting course with improvements during periods of rest from heavy weightbearing activity.

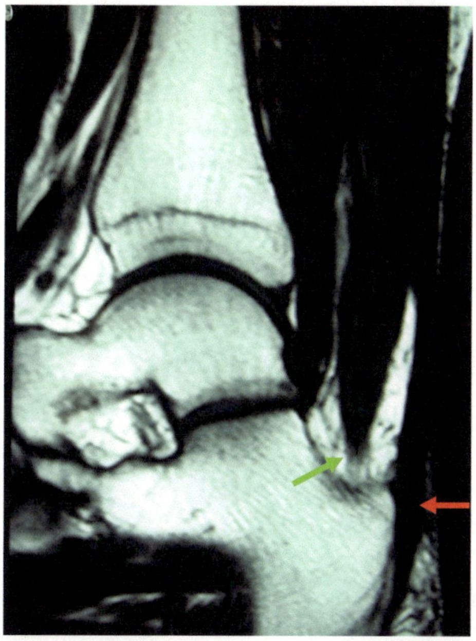

Fig. 2. MRI sagittal image of an accessory soleus muscle (green arrow) that is easily differentiated from the Achilles tendon (red arrow). The space occupying effect of this accessory soleus muscle can mimic symptoms of Achilles tendinopathy but also the features of posterior ankle impingement.

Referring to the work of Blazina et al, initially there may be pain in the tendon with the onset of weightbearing activity such as running, but the tendon pain resolves with continued running (the tendon "warms"). As the Achilles tendinopathy worsens, there may be aching after activity. With increasing use and tendon degeneration the pain may continue during the course of all weightbearing activity and may eventually preclude heavy weightbearing activity due to the level of pain. Morning pain and stiffness is a common feature of Achilles tendinopathy. Achilles tendon swelling may be noted by the patient, but it is rare to have mechanical symptoms or instability. History should ascertain if there have been any previous lower limb injuries, especially to the ankle, and also if the patient has other medical problems, is taking medication, or if there is a family history of rheumatic disease. Any treatment that the patient has had should be recorded and also if these treatments assisted with the symptoms or not.

4.2 Examination

On examination the examination should generally proceed in a structured manner to assess for the correct diagnosis, appropriate risk factors, and signs of differential diagnoses. Lower limb biomechanics should be assessed with standing and walking. In athletes it may e more appropriate to assess this with video monitoring of treadmill running or on-field training. With the patient in a standing position the examination should include assessment of foot biomechanics such as pes planus or pes cavus and subtalar hyperpronation, weightbearing ankle range of motion (ROM) including ability to perform single leg heel raise, general lower limb alignment such as genu varum or valgum, dynamic pelvic stability with Trendelenberg testing, and lumbar spine ROM and symptoms referral. Gait examination should assess for antalgic gait, reduced ankle or knee ROM, and Trendelenberg gait. With the patient sitting, perform neural tension tests such as the slump test and look for hand and nail changes of psoriasis. The patient should then be positioned supine and assessed for leg length discrepancy, lower limb neurology, and joint ROM (this must include assessment of ankle joint, subtalar joint, and 1st metatarsophlangeal (MTP) joint, but should also include assessment of knee and hip joint ROM) laxity, especially lateral ankle laxity with anterior drawer test for anterior talofibular ligament (ATFL) laxity and talar tilt test for calcaneofibular (CF) ligament laxity. Ankle plantarflexion and dorsiflexion strength, as well as 1st MTP joint flexion and extension strength, and also foot eversion and inversion strength should be assessed. Tinel's test over the tarsal tunnel and medial calcaneal nerves can be performed in the supine position. The patient may then be positioned prone for inspection of calf muscle bulk and tone, as well as any Achilles or retroAchilles swelling. Swelling and tendon thickening may be obvious either at the Achilles insertion, where bursitis or calcaneal bony protruberences may occur, or 4-6 cms proximal to this at the classic site of non-insertional Achilles tendinopathy (Figure 3).

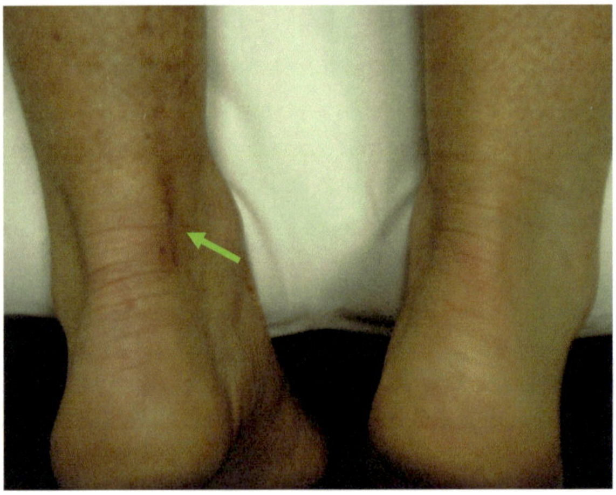

Fig. 3. The clinical manifestation of non-insertional Achilles tendinopathy is indicated by the arrow. There is obvious tendon thickening in the region 4-6 centimetres from the calcaneal insertion when compared with the other side, and this area will be tender to palpation. The tenderness may be reduced with the tendon placed under stretch by passive ankle dorsiflexion and re-palpation (London test).

Tenderness will generally be well localized to these two sites and tenderness may be reduced by placing the tendon under stretch with passive ankle dorsiflexion (London test). An assessment of tendon gliding function and crepitis may be performed in cases on non-insertional Achilles tendinopathy. Palpation of the retroAchilles space should be performed to assess for tenderness immediately deep to the distal Achilles tendon suggestive of retrocalcaneal bursitis, fullness or tenderness within the space suggestive of posterior ankle impingement, accessory soleus muscle, or other space occupying lesion. Palpation should also be performed over the tibialis posterior tendons medially and peroneal tendons laterally and strength testing performed particularly with regard to assessing for peroneal tendon subluxation or dislocation. Posterior ankle impingement sign should be checked, and calcaneal squeeze test performed to exclude calcaneal stress fracture.

This examination should allow the examiner to determine with confidence the presence or absence of Achilles tendinopathy, the site of Achilles tendinopathy and any associated features, intrinsic and intrinsic risk factors, and also exclude the common differential diagnoses for posterior heel pain.

5. Investigations

Achilles tendinopathy is essentially a clinical diagnosis and investigations are generally only required to exclude other pathology around the ankle or calf. Xrays may delineate bony or joint problems such as acute or stress fractures, os trigonum, or tarsal coalition, and may show the presence of tendon calcification that should alert the clinician to suspicion or rheumatic or metabolic disease. Lateral ankle Xray may also be used to assess for Haglund's deformity which may be associated with insertional Achilles tendinopathy. Blood tests for rheumatic disease and urate levels may be considered. Magnetic resonance Imaging (MRI) is an excellent investigation for showing the presence or absence of soft-tissue pathology around the ankle and will generally delineate Achilles tendon pathology.

Asymptomatic tendon degeneration is common and should be considered when performing any investigation on the Achilles tendon. With either ultrasound (Figure 4) or MRI the Achilles tendon ultrastructure can be assessed for tendon fusiform thickening, fibre disruption, and fluid within or around the tendon, including bursitis. These investigation findings should be accurately correlated with the site of clinical examination findings before ascribing the diagnosis and classification of Achilles tendinopathy. Doppler ultrasound is an

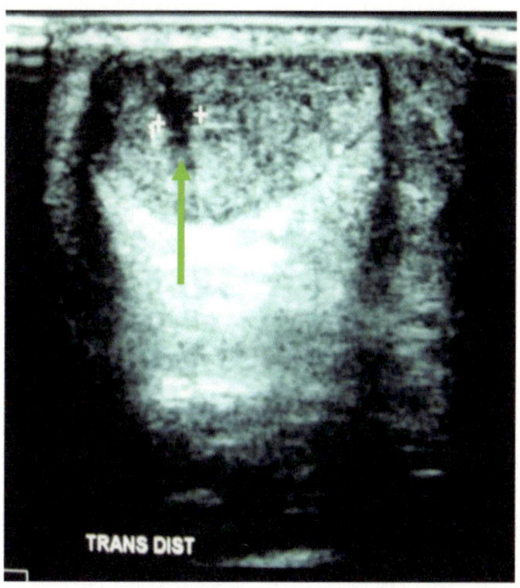

Fig. 4. Ultrasound image showing an Achilles tendon partial tear with hypoechoic region (green arrow).

extremely useful adjunct investigation for Achilles tendinopathy and may show neovascularisation, or active bursitis. Note that in the early stages of symptoms there may be no changes noted on investigation.

6. Non-surgical management of achilles tendinopathy

Treatment of all musculoskeletal injuries can involve non-surgical or surgical therapies. Non-surgical management of Achilles tendinopathy, whether insertional or non-insertional, is similar and generally involves symptom control, correction of risk factors, stretching and exercise rehabilitation, and therapeutic injections. Correction of intrinsic and extrinsic risk factors is a critical element of management to assist in decreasing abnormal load on the Achilles tendon, decreasing symptoms, and minimizing the risk of recurrence. Grading of tendinopathies is not generally clinically useful, however partial tears in the Achilles tendon will often take longer for symptoms to resolve. It is commonly stated that insertional Achilles tendinopathy is more recalcitrant to treatment, and this may be due to traction effects and calcification at the insertion (Figure 5).

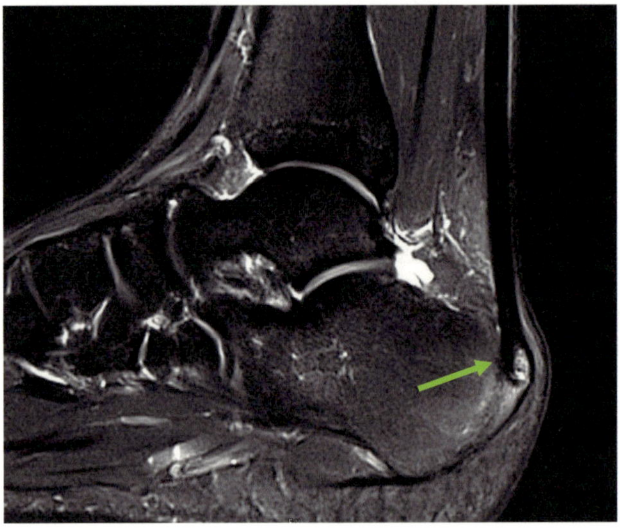

Fig. 5. Insertional Achilles tendinopathy is often more recalcitrant to treatment than non-insertional Achilles tendinopathy, and this may be due to traction effects and calcification at the insertion (green arrow). Note the bony oedema adjacent to the tendon insertion. Discrete foci of calcification may require debridement surgery if symptoms persist despite non-surgical therapies.

6.1 Symptom control

Pain is generally the dominant symptom in Achilles tendinopathy and may be managed using regular icepack application 15 minutes per time throughout the day. This may be particularly effective after exercise. Physical therapy treatment with electrotherapeutic modalities such as therapeutic ultrasound or interferential treatment may assist in decreasing pain, as may gentle transverse friction massage. Relative rest is preferred and this involves the avoidance of all aggravating activities, where possible. An aggravating activity includes any activity that cause tendon pain during the activity, tendon pain after the activity, or increased tendon pain and stiffness the morning after an activity. To avoid aggravating activites it may be necessary to avoid weightbearing exercise and to cross-train with painfree non-weightbearing exercise such as cycling, rowing/ kayaking, or swimming. Analgesics can be used to control strong pain and paracetamol/ acetaminophen is the preferred analgesic. Non-steroidal anti-inflammatory drugs (NSAIDs) should only be used where the condition is inflammatory in nature. The use of NSAIDs should be considered in early symptoms of Achilles tendon pain (the initial 2-3 weeks of symptoms), although it is uncommon for patients to present for medical care at this stage of symptoms. NSAIDs are more commonly used where bursitis, retrocalcaneal or retroAchilles, is associated with insertional Achilles tendinopathy or where paratenonitis is demonstrated to be associated with non-insertional Achilles tendinopathy. Topical agents will be discussed later in the chapter.

6.2 Correction of intrinsic risk factors

6.2.1 Biomechanics of the lower limb

Intrinsic risk factors such as lower limb biomechanical issues can generally be corrected through the use of shoes or orthotics and referral for podiatric assessment may be required. The critical element of correcting biomechanical issues is to achieve sustained control of the hindfoot. Good quality supportive footwear is one aspect of this but orthotic correction is imperative in patients with pes planus and also those with functional hyperpronation (Figure 6).

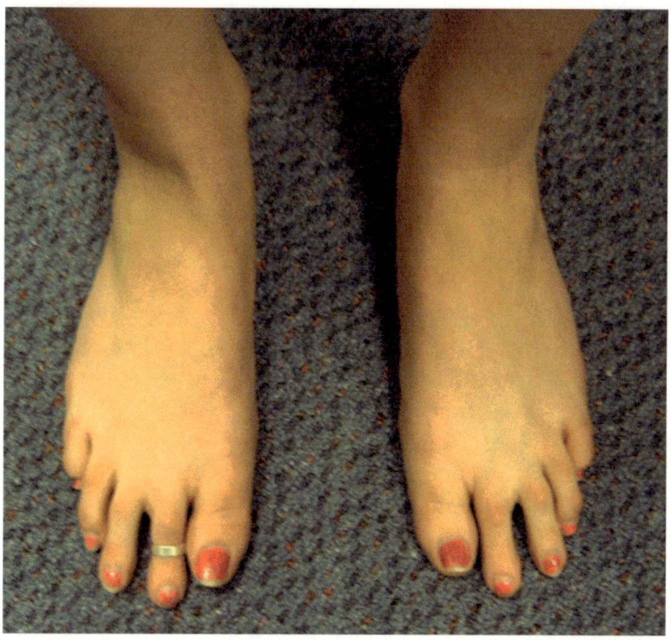

Fig. 6. Photograph of a female with subtalar hyperpronation in stance phase. Note the prominence of the medial aspect of the arch. Also note the long second toe (Morton's foot type).

Taping the handfoot and assessing the response to a patient's pain is one way to determine if orthotic prescription is likely to be beneficial for the patient. Assessing the shoes for abnormal wear patterns and for friction over the Achilles tendon is also important to determine possible causative factors in the patient's symptoms. Wedged lift heel raise devices are advocated to unload the Achilles tendon through simple biomechanical processes, but these do not control the hindfoot. Heel lift wedges should be worn at all times early in the treatment of Achilles tendinopathy and must be worn in both shoes to avoid asymmetry in gait. Any recognized leg length discrepancy over 1 cm should be corrected through built up orthotics or shoes. Before correcting this it is suggested that a more accurate determination of leg length difference is performed and a single shot scout Computerised Tomography (CT) scan can better determine this using digital calipers.

6.2.2 Joint asymmetry

Restrictions in joint range of motion can also lead to disturbance of the kinetic chain and create force imbalance between sides. The major joints that require assessment are the 1st metatrophalangeal (MTP) joint, midtarsal joints, subtalar joint, ankle joint, knee joint and hip joint. Any restriction in joint range of motion can potentially increase the load on the Achilles tendon and range of motion exercises as well as active and passive joint mobilization is required as therapy. 1st MTP joint stiffness is commonly found in patients with Achilles tendinopathy and, again, may contribute to the onset of the condition or is caused by the condition. Stretching the 1st MTP and massage through the central plantar fascia can assist in normalizing joint range of motion, but toe flexion exercises should also be incorporated into the treatment program to ensure adequate 1st MTP joint strength and endurance as this is a critical aspect of the gait cycle with 1st MTP joint flexion largely contributing to the push-off phase of walking or running.

In athletes, especially those performing unilateral upper body movements, such as tennis players, volleyball players, or throwing athletes, it is important to assess shoulder range of motion, and also trunk and thoracic spine range of motion in rotation.

6.2.3 Joint instability

There are two causes of joint instability, hereditary such as with generalized liagmentous laxity, and traumatic. Generalized liagmentous laxity is a recognized hereditary predisposition to joint laxity and is characterized by knee recurvatum, lumbar spine ligamentous laxity (as can be demonstrated by the patient being able to stand and forward flex the lumbar spine to place their palms onto the floor), laxity in elbow joints with hyperextension, and laxity in finger and thumb metacarpophalangeal (MCP) joints (demonstrated by 5th finger MCP joint extension beyond 90 degrees, and by flexing the wrist and then touching the thumb to the volar aspect of the forearm) as per Beighton's criteria. Traumatic instability to joints distal to the Achilles tendon in the kinetic chain are generally more commonly identified contributing risk factors than joints proximal to the Achilles tendon. These joints and joint injuries include the 1st metatarsophalangeal joint and 1st toe flexor dysfunction, and the ankle joint and previous lateral ligament sprains and peroneal tendon weakness, or peroneal tendon subluxation/ dislocation. Essentially, both joint laxity and joint instability contribute to the causation of Achilles tendinopathy by increasing load onto the Achilles as a the primary ankle plantarflexor, or increasing the necessity of the Achilles tendon acting to assist as an ankle joint stabilizer. Often strengthening exercise is effective as therapy for joint instability to control joint motion, but in cases of gross laxity with functional instability, such as with peroneal tendon subluxation/ dislocation, surgery may be necessary to restore joint stability and function.

6.2.4 Rheumatic and metabolic disease

Patients with hereditary rheumatic diseases such as rheumatoid arthritis or psoriatic arthritis may have tendon abnormalities manifesting as part of the systemic disease process. In rheumatoid arthritis these tend to be nodular Achilles tendon abnormalities, whereas in psoriatic arthropathy the Achilles tendon manifestation is more likely to be exuberant tendon calcification, particularly adjacent to the Achilles tendon insertion. Metabolic diseases can also present with tendon manifestations such as the crystal deposition of gout, or the lipid tendon xanthomata associated with familial hypercholesterolaemia. These systemic diseases cannot truly be cured, and the management of the tendon manifestations is through control of the generalized disease process. Large tendon nodules or xanthomata may need surgical excision to restore appropriate gliding function of the Achilles tendon.

6.3 Correction of extrinsic risk factors

6.3.1 Training errors

One of the most common extrinsic risk factors for Achilles tendinopathy in active people is training errors. This often comes do to a lack of knowledge of basic training principles such as adequate warm-up and stretching before exercise, graded increases in training, adequate recovery time through rest days, and appropriate cross-training . A key aspect of preventing injury in sports is to have adequate warm-up and stretch prior to exercise. This ensures that the musculotendinous units are at an appropriate functional length and this should allow for exercise with minimal risk of injury. Specifically for the Achilles tendon it is essential that stretching is performed for both the gastrocnemius and soleus components of the calf musculature and this would normally take the form of a straight knee calf stretch and a bent knee calf stretch.

With any level of exercise or training it is generally rapid alterations to the training program that lead to overload or overuse injuries and this is no different for Achilles tendinopathy. Common changes would include increasing the duration or frequency of training sessions, and thus the total training volume or load, but it may also be that changes occur in the intensity of training. Cross-training with different forms of exercise, including non-weightbearing exercise, can be a useful aspect of training programs but must be performed with caution in athletes not familiar with weightbearing training (i.e. swimmers that beginning running for fitness). Starting training or exercise after being sedentary is a common history in patients with Achilles tendinopathy. For this same reason, resuming training after an absence, including an enforced absence due to injury or as part of the treatment for Achilles tendinopathy, requires careful planning to ensure that the training is not too much too soon. A recurrence Achilles tendinopathy can be avoided with simple advice and planning on resumption of exercise.

6.3.2 Surfaces and equipment

Weightbearing exercise on certain surfaces may contribute to the causation of Achilles tendinopathy. Hard surfaces increase the required shock absorption for the lower limb musculotendinous structures, including the Achilles tendon, whilst soft or unstable surfaces like soft sand require the Achilles and other stabilizing tendons to increase their workload during exercise. Certainly, it is recognized that changes in the surface on which weightbearing exercise is performed can contribute to the aetiology of Achilles tendinopathy. This can be from hard to soft surfaces or vice versa, from sprung flooring to unsprung flooring, or from treadmill running to road running. In the same way, changes to exercise on hills, or on slopes or cambered surfaces can also contribute to the development of Achilles tendinopathy. This may be caused by simple changes in running routes or by beginning to run on cambered roads rather than flat running tracks. Changes in running footwear may contribute to causation in Achilles tendinopathy due to different properties of the shoes such as level of foot control or shock absorption. All of these factors should be investigated in the history and addressed in management of Achilles tendinopathy.

6.3.3 Nutrition

Fatigue is often cited as a potential cause of tendinopathy and may contribute through loss of joint or muscle control leading to increased forces acting on the Achilles tendon. Ensuring adequate hydration and energy availability to working muscle during exercise is critical to minimizing fatigue. Again, simple preparation should ensure that adequate fluid intake and carbohydrate intake is maintained before, during, and after exercise.

6.3.4 Medications

Certain medications may affect tendon metabolism and it is important to address previous and current medications to ensure that these medications are used only if absolutely necessary. Flouroquinolones such as the antibiotic ciprofloxacin have been implicated in Achilles tendon ruptures and appear to have a detrimental affect on tendon metabolism. Anabolic steroids have also been suggested as a cause of tendon rupture, possibly due to the rapid increase in muscle strength before the tendon has completed its strength adaptations. Anabolic steroids are illegal in many countries but their use is widespread nonetheless and this needs to be addressed in taking a history from the patient.

6.4 Exercise rehabilitation for achilles tendinopathy

6.4.1 Stretching

Exercise rehabilitation through muscle stretching and eccentric exercise is accepted as the mainstay of therapy for Achilles tendinopathy. The timeframe of recovery for symptom resolution in Achilles tendinopathy is in the order of 2-3 months at a minimum and both the patient and the medical practitioner need to appreciate this timeframe and commit to treatment over this period. Although stretching is advocated by most medical practitioners as part of the treatment regime, very little evidence is available to support this, or to determine the best form of stretching in treating Achilles tendinopathy. Despite this, logic would suggest that the aims of treatment with stretching are to restore musculotendinous unit length and thus static prolonged stretching should best achieve this aim. Stretching both the gastrocnemius muscle, through straight knee calf stretching, and also the soleus muscle component, through flexed knee calf stretching, is important to ensure that all components of the Achilles musculotendinous unit are incorporated in the stretching program. Stretching to the point of pain is generally discouraged and, especially in insertional Achilles tendinopathy, may be counterproductive and continue to irritate the symptoms and prolong recovery time. Any recognized muscle asymmetry also requires correction through stretching and a general lower limb stretching program should be considered. The kinetic chain relationship between the 1st metatarsophalangeal joint in toe flexion with toe "push-off" and the Achilles musculotendinous unit as an ankle plantarflexor and stabilizer in this gait phase is appreciated and requires that 1st metatarsophalangeal joint range of motion is optimal to assist in managing load through the Achilles tendon. Thus, stretching the 1st metatarsophalangeal joint is a critical part of management of Achilles tendinopathy.

6.4.2 Exercise rehabilitation

Again it is worth emphasizing that exercise rehabilitation through muscle stretching and eccentric exercise is accepted as the mainstay of therapy for Achilles tendinopathy. Numerous studies have demonstrated the symptom reduction achieved through eccentric exercise protocols in Achilles tendinopathy. Irrespective of other treatments used or considered in the treatment of Achilles tendinopathy, eccentric exercise must form an integral part of the treatment program in this condition.

Tensile loading of musculotendinous units stimulates tendon healing along appropriate lines and directions of force and allows the tendons to achieve the necessary strength and endurance required to accept loading with weightbearing activity. This tensile loading appears to be best achieved through eccentric exercise protocols. The type of eccentric exercise is similar for both insertional and non-insertional Achilles tendinopathy but the range of motion in the eccentric phase differs to achieve the best symptom reduction in each specific type of Achilles tendinopathy. Alfredson et al (Alfredson , 1998) demonstrated that eccentric exercise is effective in reducing pain in Achilles tendinopathy and is as effective as surgical treatment for symptom reduction (Figure 7). This group showed that heavy-load eccentric exercise could reduce pain levels form an average of 7 out of 10 to an average of 3 out of 10. It is important to recognize that few patients became completely asymptomatic with this treatment regime alone.The eccentric exercise involved heel-drop exercises off a step, with the forefoot only on the step and, as would be expected, two forms of eccentric exercise were used, one with the knee flexed and one with the knee straight in order to load both the soleus and gastrocnemius components of the Achilles musculotendinous unit. The protocol of heavy-load eccentric exercise used in this landmark study involved twice daily heel-drop exercises with three sets of 15 repetitions with a flexed knee and three sets of 15 repetitions with a flexed knee. This is a combined total of 180 heel drop exercises. This protocol is time consuming but is recognized as the appropriate level of eccentric exercise required to achieve a symptom reducing effect. It is critical to note that there is no active concentric, or muscle shortening, phase of the exercise and recovery of ankle position needs to be assisted either by weightberaing on the other leg or, preferably, by using the arms to pull up on a stair rail or other fixed structure to recover ankle position. Neisen-Vertommen et al (Neisen-Vertommen, 1992) further demonstrated that eccentric exercise alone was more effective the concentric-eccentric exercise and this is the reason that it is important to minimize, or.

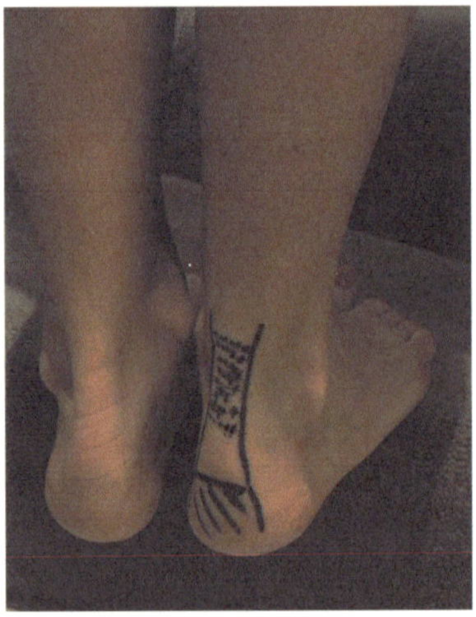

Fig. 7. Eccentric heel drop exercises using a stair or step. The forefoot is on the step with the midfoot and hindfoot unsupported. The heel is then lowered and an eccentric exercises component will generated (tendon lengthening under load). This eccentric exercise is the core component of exercise therapy for Achilles tendinopathy.

abolish, any active concentric exercise component in the heel-drop exercise rehabilitation. Eccentric exercise rehabilitation for non-insertional Achilles tendinopathy should be performed is a slow and controlled manner and the heel should generally reach below the horizontal level of the step With the knee flexed, the heel will not reach far below this horizontal level. There is no benefit from holding the exercise at this end-range as the presumed benefit of eccentric exercise is the tensile lengthening of the musculotendinous unit under weightbearing load. Recent research suggests that in the treatment of insertional tendinopathy the heel drop exercises should be performed is a slow and controlled manner and the heel should not reach below the horizontal level of the step. This may allow for the tensile forces to act on the musculotendinous unit whilst also minimizing the traction effect on the Achilles tendon insertion.

6.5 Topical medications

6.5.1 Topical glyceryl trinitrate

Glyceryl trinitrate has a long history of therapeutic use, being discovered as an effective treatment of angina pectoris in miners handling the explosive nitroglycerin in the 1870's. The mechanism of action of topical glyceryl trinitrate is suggested to be through the biologically active metabolite nitric oxide, also termed endothelial derived relaxing factor, due to the vasodilatory action of this metabolite. In animal studies, the addition of nitric oxide to injured tendon was demonstrated to improve tendon healing, although the exact mechanism of this action is not clear. It may be an analgesic effect, an effect on global tendon bloodflow, or an effect on the tendon neovessels seen as a histopathologic response in degenerative tendinopathy. As a result of the basic science research into topical glyeryl trinitrate, studies were performed to assess the effect of topical glyeryl trinitrate in symptom reduction in non-insertional Achilles tendinopathy [Paoloni, 2004]. This randomized controlled clinical trial demonstrated significant pain reduction, increase in object tendon strength measures, and an increased rate of patients being completely asymptomatic after six months of treatment. The topical glyeryl trinitrate was applied as a patch (Figure 8) over the symptomatic tender area of the Achilles tendon and was used in continuous dosage.

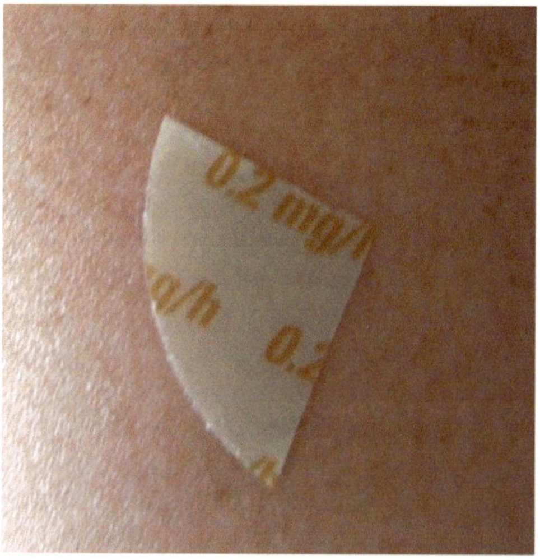

Fig. 8. The topical glyceryl trinitrate patch used in clinical trials to effectively treat the symptoms of non-insertional Achilles tendinopathy. This patch is one quarter of a 5mg/ 24 hour (0.2 mg/ hour) NitroDur® patch (manufactured by Schering-Plough Australia), howver similar drug dosages can be achieved with other glyceryl trinitrate patches or ointments.

The continuous dosage regime was designed to minimize the frequency and severity of side-effects through tolerance to the vascular side-effects of the patch, as opposed to the "drug holiday" regime used in cardiovascular medicine where there is a need to maintain vascular sensitivity to nitric oxide to ensure adequate vasodilatation. The side-effects of topical glyeryl trinitrate include headache and rash and approximately 5-10% of patients will not tolerate the patch usage to treat Achilles tendinopathy due to these problematic, but reversible, side-effects. It must be emphasized that the topical glyeryl trinitrate treatment is used in addition to exercise rehabilitation. Topical glyceryl trinitrate treatment, especially continuously, is contraindicated in patients with known cardiovascular disease, especially angina pectoris, due to the potential development of tolerance to topical glyceryl trinitrate vasodilatation effects.

6.5.2 Topical anti-inflammatory medications

As symptom relief is an important aspect of the treatment of Achilles tendinopathy, there may be a role for topical anti-inflammatory medications to treat Achilles tendinopathy, especially insertional Achilles tendinopathy associated with retrocalcaneal or retroAchilles bursitis. These topical anti-inflammatory agents may take the form of non-steroidal anti-inflammatory drugs (NSAIDs) such as diclofenac or piroxicam creams, or may be other medications such as traumeel®, an interesting semi-homeopathic preparation containing measurable amounts of multiple natural substances such as arnica and Echinacea, and having shown evidence of anti-inflammatory properties mainly in treating gastrointestinal disorders.

6.6 Injection therapies in achilles tendinopathy

6.6.1 Corticosteroid and anti-inflammatory injections

Corticosteroids are catabolic steroids that have anti-inflammatory properties and are widely used in musculoskeletal medicine. In weightbearing tendons, such as the Achilles or patellar tendon, there is a theoretical risk of tendon rupture after corticosteroid injections. This may be due to the catabolic effect of corticosteroids, with a transient weakening of tendon substance, it may be due to the incorrect placement of the injection into the tendon substance creating pressure necrosis and catabolic effects, or it may be due to the pre-existing degenerative process in the tendon that has already weakened the tendon substance. Few studies have assessed the effect of corticosteroids in the treatment of Achilles tendinopathy, however one study [Da Cruz, 1988] using ultrasound guided corticosteroid injection into the Achilles paratenon in non-insertional Achilles tendinopathy did not show any statistically significant improvement. This may be due to the degenerative nature of the pathologic process in chronic Achilles tendinopathy, although it is conceivable that this treatment may be effective in the first few weeks of symptoms of Achilles tendon pain, when an acute inflammatory response may be present. Corticosteroid injections may be more useful as therapeutic agents where retrocalcaneal bursitis (Figure 9) or retroAchilles bursitis is present with insertional Achilles tendinopathy. The indications for using corticosteroid injections are generally for decreasing severe pain to allow the patient to perform exercise rehabilitation relatively pain free, or when there is a plateau in any improvement with exercise rehabilitation. These injections are best performed guided to minimize the risk of intratendinous injection and thus potential tendon rupture. With ultrasound visualisation the fluid in the distended bursa may be seen, under Doppler ultrasound increased vascularity in the bursa may be appreciated, and the injection can also be seen to be in the bursa with bursal filling demonstrated.

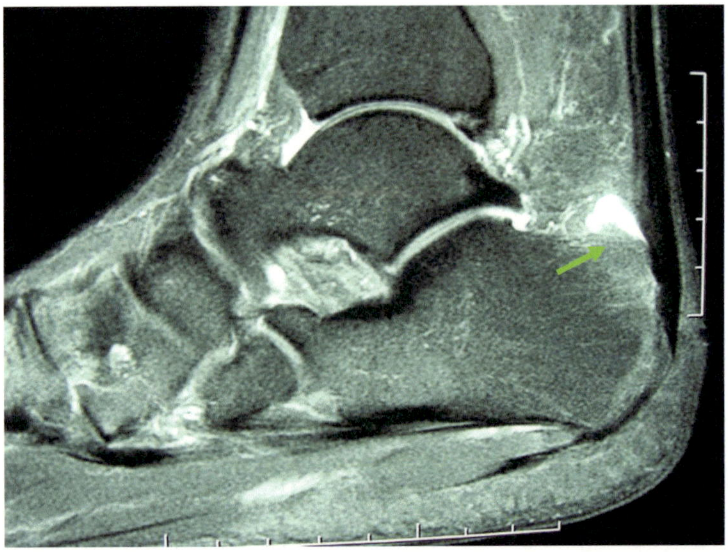

Fig. 9. MRI sagittal image showing retrocalcaneal bursitis (arrow). This may be effectively treated using injected corticosteroid agents.

Where there is a suggestion that pain is potentially caused by inflammation, such as in non-insertional Achilles peritenonitis or where the pain is at the level 4-6 cms above the tendon insertion but there are nil ultrastructural changes or abnormal vascularity in this region, or at the Achilles insertion with associated retrocalcaneal or retroAchilles bursitis, and there is a concern about possible tendon rupture with the catabolic effect of corticosteroid injection, then other anti-inflammatory agents such as traumeel® injection may be considered. This may be the case where active patients or athletes will not be able to unload the tendon after injection. Any symptom relieving effect of traumeel® injection in this circumstance may be due to a dilution effect of any chemical irritation at the site of pain.

6.6.2 Polidocanol sclerotherapy injections

Polidocanol is a sclerosant medication that has predominantly been used to treat venous varicosities. However, studies have demonstrated a positive therapeutic effect in treating Achilles tendinopathy through the use of Doppler ultrasound guided polidocanol injections [Ohberg, 2002], and this effect appears to persist at 2 year follow-up[Lind, 2006]. Ohberg et al reported that the pain reducing effect was in the order of 80% pain reduction in approximately 80% of patients when using between one and five guided polidocanol injection sessions. The procedure involves assessing the Achilles tendon for increased vascularity under Doppler ultrasound, compared to normal tendon substance that does not show any vasuclarity under Doppler ultrasound (Figure 10). The vascularity is believed to be due to neovascularisation, part of the pathologic process of degenerative tendinopathy. It is relatively common to view a single vessel, or a few vessels, entering the tendon from the deep aspect and then branching more widely throughout the tendon substance. To avoid pressure necrosis it is best to attempt to sclerose the vessels at the tendon undersurface and use as small an amount of polidocanol sclerosant as is possible. The more accurately the needle tip can be visualized the better the sclerosant effect and the less infiltrate that will be

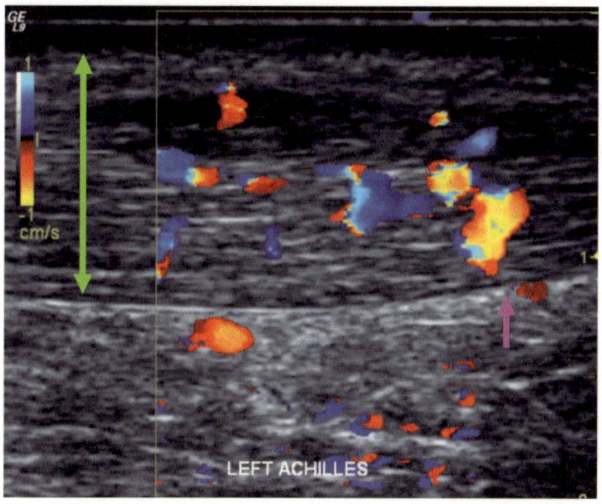

Fig. 10. Colour Doppler ultrasound image showing the Achilles tendon (green arrow marks the Achilles tendon) with thickening of the tendon, a hypoechoic region suggestive of small partial tendon tear, and prominent vascularity. The vascularity often appears to enter from the undersurface of the tendon (pink arrow) and then branch through the tendon. Sclerosing the vascularity at the entry point to the tendon can be an effective treatment for symptom reduction.

required during the procedure. This takes experience but should allow immediate abolition of the vascularity in the tendon as visualized in real-time under Doppler ultrasound. The effect can be quite impressive, but is not always complete. Repeating the procedure may be required if pain is not decreased or abolished. As reported in the initial study on polidocanol sclerotherapy [Ohberg, 2002], it may take several injections to achieve adequate symptom resolution. There does not appear to be any negative effect on tendon structure with polidocanol injections and the tendon may be loaded normally within a few days after the injection without any apparent risk. If bursitis is found to be associated with increased tendon vascularity, then it is recommended that polidocanol injections be used to sclerose the neovessels and corticosteroid is infiltrated into the inflamed bursa during the same ultrasound procedure. This may then require 5-7 days of rest before returning to normal tendon loading, in order to allow the corticosteroid to have an effect on the bursal inflammation.

6.6.3 Prolotherapy injections

Prolotherapy, or "proliferation therapy", is a term that is generally applied to various non-pharmacologic injection types all of which are proposed to act to strengthen weakened degenerative connective tissue in tendon presumably by an irritant effect. There are mostly used at insertions of tendons or ligaments. The types of solutions vary but commonly used injection types include glucose, local anesthetics such as lidocaine, phenol, or glycerine. In most medical practices it is the relatively innocuous injections such as glucose and lidocaine that are used due to the low side-effect profile. Prolotherapy injections may be considered, after weighing the risks and benefits of these, for recalcitrant insertional Achilles tendinopathy. Again, a period of rest is probably required after the injection and then continuance of exercise rehabilitation program.

6.6.4 Autologous blood product injections

Autologous blood products have been used as injection therapy in musculoskeletal medicine for many decades. This may be in the form of autologous blood or as blood extracts such as platelet rich plasma (PRP) or isolated specific growth factors such as fibroblast growth factor or platelet derived growth factor. The therapeutic use of isolated growth factors for specific musculoskeletal injury is still in its infancy, and is currently prohibited for competitive athletes under the World Anti-Doping Authority (WADA) code January, 2011. The evidence for the use of autologous blood products, including platelet rich plasma, to treat Achilles tendinopathy or other tendinopathies is scant and most well conducted clinical trials do not show evidence of effect [de Vos, 2010 and Paoloni, 2010]. However many facets of the use of these injections have not been established, including; what is the optimal blood product injection type, what is the optimal volume of injection, what is the optimal timing of injection after injury, what is the optimal number and spacing of injections (single injection versus injection series, and what the optimal rehabilitation is after injection. These autologous blood product injections are probably best used for cases of recalcitrant insertional Achilles tendinopathy where they may have an irritant or proliferative effect similar to that of prolotherapy injections. The risks and benefits need to be weighed before deciding on these injections, but the side-effect profile is low, with post-injection pain and irritation for up to 1-2 weeks the most likely side-effect. The irritant side-effects may be greater if these products are injected into the tendon substance rather than around the tendon.

6.6.5 Mesotherapy injections

Mesotherapy is widely practiced in sports medicine and refers to the use of multiple injections, often of anti-inflammatory medications such as piroxicam, into the subcutaneous fat overlying a region of musculoskeletal pain. The evidence for this treatment is also scant and the mechanism of effect appears unclear but may be due to localised tissue uptake of anti-inflammatory medication. This treatment may provide symptomatic relief especially in insertional Achilles tendinopathy associated with retrocalcaneal or retoAchilles bursitis. Mesotherapy is generally performed as a series of three sessions of multiple subcutaneous injections over a three week period.

7. Surgical treatment for achilles tendinopathy

Surgical treatment for Achilles tendinopathy is generally reserved for recalcitrant cases where non-surgical management has failed to provide effective symptom relief or ability to function in daily life or in sporting activities. It is often dictated by the patient who may become frustrated by continued symptoms despite long periods of exercise rehabilitation and also trials of injections and other therapies. It is reported that between 24% and 46% of patients with Achilles tendinopathy eventually require some form of surgical treatment, however this rates appears quite high and may represent the incidence of surgery in patients presenting to orthopaedic surgeons [Maffulli, 2002]. Many patients with Achilles tendinopathy may never consult a surgical specialist for their condition. It must be recognised that probably 10-20% of patients with Achilles tendinopathy continue to have symptoms in the longer term and it is this population that would be considered for surgical treatment. Conditions such as chronic bursitis, especially associated with Haglund's deformity, may require surgery (Figure 11).

7.1 Tendon surgery

The exact surgical procedure used to treat Achilles tendinopathy varies amongst surgeons and geographical regions but will generally involve; tendon debridement and bursal resection, if required. The tendon debridement may take the form of multiple longitudinal incisions into the Achilles tendon substance with or without curettage of any mucoid degenerative areas, or may be less invasive and involve debridement of the tendon surface and paratenon only. Any bursal involvement at the Achilles insertion should warrant bursal resection. The majority of patients will experience symptom reduction after surgery, 85% of patients report good results after surgery, and many patients will be able to return to previous level of activities or sport within six to twelve months post-surgery whether surgery is performed with open procedures [Saxena, 2003] or less invasive methods [Maffull, 1997].

7.2 Surgery procedures for bony abnormalities

There may be bony abnormalities that contribute to the development of Achilles tendinopathy and these may nee to be addressed surgically. Surgery may be only to rectify these bony abnormalities or it may be in combination with tendon debridement surgery.

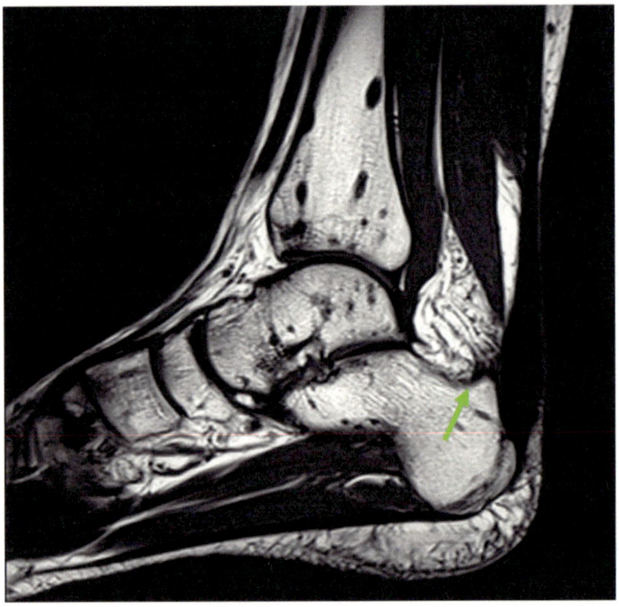

Fig. 11. Chronic fat pad inflammation, Haglund's deformity (arrow) and insertional Achilles tendinopathy. This case may require surgery for ongoing symptoms. Also note the osteopoikilosis, a benign condition manifesting as dark bone islands on MRI.

Haglund's deformity is a posterosuperior bony calcaneal protruberance that may predispose to both retrocalcaneal bursitis and to insertional Achilles tendinopathy due to a mechanical friction effect on the deep surface of the Achilles tendon (Figure 8). If Haglund's deformity is present and there is concomitant recalcitrant Achilles tendinopathy then it may be necessary to perform surgical excision of the Haglund's deformity. Sever hindfoot abnormalities with hindfoot varus may also predispose to Achilles tendinopathy through a twisting or "wringing out" mechanism of the collagen fibres and microvasculature. Correction of moderate flexible hindfoot varus caused by subtalar hyperpronation may be achieved through footwear and orthotics as discussed earlier, however severe hindfoot varus or fixed hindfoot varus may require surgical correction through calcaneal osteotomy or similar biomechanic realignment procedures.

8. Conclusion

The aetiology of Achilles tendinopathy is complex and multifactorial and the management of this condition requires a thorough understanding of the extrinsic and extrinsic risks factors, biomechanics or the lower limb and the concept of the kinetic chain. Management of Achilles tendinopathy, whether insertional or non-insertional, should always be non-surgical initially, and must focus on elements of pain control, correction of intrinsic and extrinsic risk factors, and exercise rehabilitation through appropriate stretching and eccentric exercise protocols. Other modalities such as topical or injected medications may be required if pain is not controlled or if symptomatic improvement with exercise rehabilitation plateaus. Based on stratification of risks and benefits in patients with recalcitrant Achilles tendinopathy, and no cardiovascular disease, a sensible approach to adjunctive modalities would start with topical agents such as continuous topical glyceryl trinitrate treatment in addition to exercise rehabilitation. Further adjunctive treatment with injections differs depending on the site of Achilles tendinopathy. In both insertional and non-insertional Achilles tendinopathy, an assessment of the tendon is made using ultrasound and Doppler mode. For patients with either insertional or non-insertional Achilles tendinopathy who demonstrate increases in vascularity in the tendon substance at the site that correlates with symptoms, Doppler ultrasound guided polidocanol injections should be the first-line treatment to assist in alleviating symptoms. Should there be ultrastructural tendon abnormalities without increased tendon vascularity at the symptomatic tendon site in non-insertional Achilles tendinopathy, then the preferred injection treatment becomes less clear and options would include; autologous blood or platelet rich plasma (PRP) into the degenerative area of the tendon or around the tendon, or other injections around the tendon which would include traumeel®, prolotherapy type agents such as glucose or lidocaine, or indeed innocuous injection agents such as normal saline.

9. Acknowledgment

This work would not have been possible without the support and encouragement of all the staff at the Orthopaedic Research Institute (ORI), St George Hospital campus, and the University of New South Wales, Australia.

10. References

Alfredson, H., Pietila, T., Jonsson, P., et al. Heavy-load eccentric calf muscle training for the treatment of chronic Achilles tendinosis. *Am J Sports Med*, Vol. 26, No. 3 (1998), pp. 360-366.

DaCruz, D., Geeson, M., Allen, M.J., et al, Achilles' paratendonitis: an evaluation of steroid injection. Am J Sports Med, Vol 22, No. 2, (1988), pp. 64-65.

Lind, B., Ohberg, L., Alfredson, H. Sclerosing polidocanol injections in mid-portion Achilles tendinosis: remaining good clinical results and decreased tendon thickness at 2-year follow-up. *Knee Surg Sport Trauma Arth.* Vol 14, No. 12 (2006), pp. 1327-1332. de Vos, R.J., Weir, A., van Schie, H.T.M., et al. Platelet-rich plasma injection for chronic Achilles tendinopathy: a randomised controlled trial. *JAMA*, Vol 303, (2010), pp. 144-149.

Maffulli, N., Kader, D.. Tendinopathy of tendo achillis. *J Bone Joint Surg [Br]*, Vol. 84 (2002), pp. 1-8.

Maffulli, N., Testa, V., Capasso, G. Results of percutaneous longitudinal tenotomy for Achilles tendinopathy in middle- and long-distance runners. *Am J Sport Med* , Vol 25 (1997), pp. 835-840.

Niesen-Vertommen, S., Taunton, J.E., Clement, D.B. The effect of eccentric versus concentric exercise in the management of Achilles tendonitis. Clin J Sports Med, Vol 2 (1992), pp. 109-113.

Ohberg, L., Alfredson, H. Ultrasound guided sclerosis of neovessels in painful chronic Achilles tendinosis: pilot study of a new treatment. *Br J Sport Med*, Vol 36, No. 3, (2002), pp. 173-177.

Paoloni, J., de Vos, R.J., Hamilton, B., et al. Platelet rich plasma treatment for ligament and tendon injuries. *Clin J Sport Med*, Vol 21, (2011), pp. 37-45.

Paoloni, J.A., Appleyard, R.C., Murrell, G.A.C. Topical Glyceryl Trinitrate Treatment of Chronic Non-insertional Achilles Tendinopathy: A Randomized, Double-Blind, Placebo Controlled Clinical Trial. *J Bone Joint Surg [Am]*, Vol 86A, No. 5 (2004), pp. 916-922.

Saxena, A., Cheung, S. Surgery for chronic Achilles tendinopathy. Review of 91 procedures over 10 years. *J Am Podiatr Med Assoc*, Vol 93, (2003), pp. 283-291.

Part 4

Achilles Tendon Ruptures

6

ABO Blood Groups and Achilles Tendon Injury

Gian Nicola Bisciotti, Cristiano Eirale and Pier Paolo Lello
Kinemove Rehabilitation Centers, Pontremoli, La Spezia, Parma
Italy

1. Introduction

The incidence of Achilles tendon rupture has significantly increased over the last 20 years (Moller, 1996; Young and Maffulli, 2007), achieving, within the tendon diseases, an incidence between 6 and 18% (Rees et al., 2006; Mazzone and McCue, 2002; Shepsis et al., 2002). The risk of the Achilles tendon rupture is greater in the male population with a ratio included between 1.7 : 1 and 30 : 1. This data would be justified by the high prevalence of males subjects in sports considered at risk (Rees et al., 2006; Mazzone and McCue). Despite its high incidence in the context of sports traumatology, the Achilles tendon rupture etiology remains poorly known (Maffulli, 1999; Williams, 1986) and it is essentially based on two main theories: the "degenerative theory" and the "mechanical theory".

The "degenerative theory

From a biomechanical point of view, the "degenerative theory" is based on the assumption that a structurally intact tendon, even if subjected to significant tensile forces - however remaining within the physiological request - should not be subject to rupture (Cetti and Christensen, 1983). In fact, since 1959 (Arnero and Lindhom, 1959), we can find in bibliography several studies showing that the majority of patients undergoing Achilles tendon surgical repair, already had rather advanced degenerative processes that were considered responsible for the tendon structural failure (Davidsson and Salo, 1969; Fox et al 1975; Kannus and Jozsa, 1991; Jozsa et al., 1991; Jarvinen, 1997; Jozsa andKannus, 1997; Waterston, 1997; Waterston and Maffulli, 1997). Although most of these degenerative involutions were not linked to a precise etiologic cause, the majority of the Authors linked these to an alteration in tendon microcirculation subsequent to hypoxia and altered metabolism (Jarvinen, 1997; Jozsa and Kannus, 1997; Waterston, 1997; Waterston and Maffulli, 1997). Others Authors noted that the degenerated tendon tissue showed an increased production of collagen type III and V that disturbs the normal architecture of the tendon tissue making it less resistant against mechanical stress (Waterston, 1997; Waterston et al., 1997).

The mechanical theory

Some Authors showed that the Achilles tendon structural failure can occur even if it is subjected to mechanical stress that is within a normal physiological situation but in a situation where the tendon was, or may be, subject to a series of cumulative microtraumatic injuries without having allowed a reasonable time for the biological repair (Knörzer et al., 1986; Selvanetti et al., 1997). Therefore, the complete rupture would be the result of a several number of previous multiple microtraumatic injuries which would lead the tendon just to the point of its structural failure (Knörzer et al., 1986). In such conditions, the situation of greater risk for the tendon integrity would occur when they are present within the same moment three very specific biomechanical factors (Barfred, 1971; Hess et al., 1989).).

- The tendon is obliquely loaded in relation to its anatomical axis.
- The gastrocnemius-soleus muscle complex is in maximal contraction.
- The initial tendon length is reduced.

We can find this combination of factors as a usual situation almost in all sports requiring a "push off" quick action (Selvanetti et al., 1997). The mechanical theory could, at least in part explain the occurrence of the Achilles tendon complete rupture as this event is sometimes observed even in the absence of degenerative processes (Knörzer et al., 1986; Clement et al., 1994). In according with this situation it is interesting to note that some Authors have suggested a relationship between the musculoskeletal disorders and in particular, tendon disorders and subjects' blood group (Mourant et al., 1978; Lourie, 1983; Joza et al., 1989; Kujala et al., 1992). The scientific rationale for this correlation is based on the fact that subjects belonging to 0 blood groups show an N-acetylgalactosamine transferase activity higher compared to subjects belonging to the A and B group (Kujala et al., 1992). A greater N-acetylgalactosamine transferase activity leads to a collagen type III increased production within the tendon (Waterston and Maffulli, 1997). The type III collagen is less resistant against mechanical stress compared to type I collagen (Waterston and Maffulli, 1997) and would predispose the tendon to spontaneous rupture (Joza et al., 1989; Maffulli, 1999). This may explain the high incidence of Achilles tendon spontaneous ruptures found by some Authors in subjects belonging to the 0 blood group compared to the A and B groups (Joza et al., 1989; Maffulli, 1999).

In addition to these two main theories, the Achilles tendon rupture may result from other different factors that we can assume as follows:

2. The iatrogenic damage

The use of corticosteroids

The use of corticosteroids are widely used therapeutic practice in a various number of diseases, however their use represents a risk factor for tendon rupture (Fisher, 2004) In literature some Authors report clear associations between rupture of the Achilles tendon and oral assumption and tendinous or peritendinous injections of corticosteroids (Unverferth and Olix, 1973; Newnham et al., 1991). The recommendation to not use corticosteroids in tendinopathy is based over two main points:

i. Their potential danger against the integrity of the tendon structure (Speed, 2001).
ii. An insufficient evidence to justify their use in tendinopathy (Maffulli and Kader, 2002).

The use of fluoroquinolone

The use of some antibiotics such as fluoroquinolone is associated in literature with injury and / or to serious tendon ruptures, especially at Achilles tendon level (Huston, 1994; Royer et al., 1994; Filippucci et al., 2003 ; Vanek et al., 2003). The first Achilles tendon rupture due to the use of fluoroquinolone was described in 1992 (Ribard et al., 1992). The fluoroquinolone are drugs widely used in clinical practice but their association with corticosteroid drugs, especially in the elderly subjects, is an important risk factor for tendinopathy and/or tendon rupture (Linden Van Der et al., 2003). The most important number of tendon damages caused by fluoroquinolone reported in the literature is caused by the use of ciprofloxacin followed by enoxacin, ofloxacin and enorfloxacin (Huston, 1994; Szarfman et al., 1995; Van der Linden et al., 2002; Filippucci et al., 2003). The fluoroquinolone-induced tendon degeneration would be due to the destruction of the extra cellular matrix, to the inhibition of tenocytes proliferation and to the reduction of collagen synthesis (Szarfman et al., 1995; Corps et al., 2003).

3. The intrinsic factors

The intrinsic factors, otherwise defined as endogenous factors, which may give rise to Achilles tendinopathy mainly concern paramorphisms or particular postural aspects that may lead to a functional overload at Achilles tendon level compromising its functionality and structure.

Among these we can mention:

The iper-pronation of the hindfoot associated or not to flat-foot (Ryan et al., 2009; Wyndow et al., 2010).

A varus forefoot associated or not to valgus hindfoot (Ajis et al, 2005)

A flat-supinated foot (Ryan et al., 2009; Wyndow et al., 2010).

A retrocalcaneal spur (Kearney and Costa, 2010)

An Haglund's deformity (Min et al., 2010)

A lower limb asymmetry (Kannus, 1997).

A limitation in ankle dorsiflexion (Kaufman et al., 1999).

A limitation of the subtalar joint mobility (Kvist, 1991).

A poor muscle strength of lower limbs in general and particularly of the calf muscles. In fact, a muscle with a stamina few level cannot effectively protects the tendon structure (Kannus, 1997).

The Dehydration (Hestin et al., 1993; Schwellnus et al., 1997; Gottschalk and Andrish, 2011).

The hyperlipidemia (Mathiak et al., 1999; Ozgurtas et al., 2003).

The hyperuricemia (Dodds e Burry, 1984).

The tendon temperature increase resulting from sporting activities (Wilson e Goodship, 1994).

Changes in the genes expression regulating the "cell-cell" and the "cell-matrix" interaction, associated to a matrix metal proteinase 3 (MMP-3) down-regulation and to a metal proteinase 2 (MMP-2) and Vascular Endothelian Growth Factor (VEGF). up-regulation (Ajis and Maffulli, 2007).

4. The extrinsic factor

In several sports, especially in those where its expected the run and/or the jumps, the injuries and / or the Achilles tendon tears are often associated with errors in the training planning (Hess et al., 1989; Clain and Baxter, 1992; Jozsa and Kannus, 1997; Mahieu et al., 2006). One of the most important causes seems represented by overtraining (Clement e coll, 1984), then follow the changes and / or the increasing in the training program carried out without an appropriate adaptation period (Kvist, 1991; Kwist, 1994; Järvinen et al., 2001) and a lack of specific athletic skill (James e coll., 1978). Others extrinsic factors that may give rise to Achilles tendinopathy that we must remember are: fatigue, poor technique, poor equipment and environment conditions (temperature, humidity, altitude, wind) (Young and Maffulli, 2007).

The aim of this study is to verify, through a retrospective analysis, conducted in an active sports population, the incidence of both Achilles tendons spontaneous ruptures and tendinopathy in relationship to the blood group.

5. Subjects

We considered two different groups composed by 45 caucasian patients belonging to the Northern Italy population whose age, weight and height was respectively 32±7 years, 78±6,7 kg and 178±5,5 cm. In the first group (G1), all subjects attended our medical center complaining of Achilles tendon pain or following a surgery of scarification or open tenorraphy at this level. G1 patients practiced sport activity at professional or amateur level. 24 patients (53,3% of the subjects) followed a conservative program for Achilles tendinopathy, while the two groups of patients surgically treated 15 subjects (equal to 33,3%), with open tenorraphy and 6 subjects, (13,3%) with tendon scarification) were following the specific post-surgery rehabilitation program. In the second group (G2) all subjects. practiced a sport activity at professional or amateur level but none of them had never suffered for tendinopathy during his career. All the subjects were informed of the aim of the study and gave their written consent for the data processing.

6. Protocols and methods

All subjects were required to produce an official document in which their blood group was annotated. The clinical diagnosis of Achilles tendinopathy, formulated for the 20 patients who had not undergone surgical treatment, was confirmed by ultrasonography performed in accordance with the criteria in the following form (Annex A). Both clinical and imaging criteria were adopted in accordance with the protocol already used by the Research Unit for Exercise Science and Sports Medicine, University of Cape Town (Schepsis et al., 2002; Alison et al., 2007; Collins et al., 2010). The clinical criteria allowing us to formulate diagnosis of Achilles tendinopathy were:

- Gradual progressive pain over the Achilles tendon area > 6 weeks
- Early morning pain
- Early morning stiffness
- History of swelling over the Achilles tendon area
- Tenderness to palpation over the Achilles tendon
- Palpable nodular thickening over the affected Achilles
- Positive "shift" test (movement of the nodular area with plantar dorsi-flexion).

7. Statistic

For all considered variables the usual statistical indices (average and standard deviation) were calculated. The normality of data distributions was checked with a Kolmorogov-Smirnov test. The difference between the recorded values and the expected values was calculated by a Chi Square Test, the statistic significance was posed to $p<0.05$.

8. Results

G1 group

30 subjects (66.6%) belonged to group 0. 19 of these 30 subjects (equal to 63.3%) had undergone a chirurgical tenorraphy, 7 subjects (equal to 23.3%) had undergone a chirurgical scarification and the remaining 4 subjects (equal to 13,3%) had undergone a conservative treatment.

8 subjects, equal to 17.7%, belonged to group A. 6 of these 8 subject (equal to 75%) had undergone a chirurgical tenorraphy and the remaining 2 subjects (equal to 25%%) had undergone a chirurgical scarification.

4 subjects equal to 8.8% belonged to B group. 2 of these 4 subjects (equal to 50%) had undergone a chirurgical tenorraphy while the remaining 2 subjects (equal to the 50%) had undergone a conservative treatment.

3 subjects equal to the 6.6% belonged to the group AB. All these subjects had undergone to a chirurgical scarification.

All subjects were male.

G2 group

18 subjects (equal to 40%) belonged to group 0.

20 subjects (equal to 44,4%) belonged to the A group.

5 subjects (equal to 11,1%) belonged to the B group.

2 subjects (equal to 4.4%) belonged to the AB group

All subjects were male.

The difference between the subjects belonged to group 0 in G1 an G2 group was statistically significant ($p<0.005$).

The difference between the subjects belonged to group A in G1 an G2 group was statistically significant ($p<0.01$).

The difference between the subjects belonged to group B in G1 an G2 group was not statistically significant.

The difference between the subjects belonged to group AB in G1 an G2 group was not statistically significant ($p<0.01$).

9. Discussion

Already in the second half of the last century (Aird et al., 1953) several works showing an association between the blood groups and different types of pathology were published. In this context, we can mention the relationship between blood groups and hip primary osteoarthritis (Lourie, 1983), acute hematogenous osteomyelitis (Eid, 1985), tendon ruptures (Jozsa et al., 1989; Kujala et al., 1992; Mafuli et al., 2000), nail-patella syndrome (Renwich and Lawler, 1955), spondylolisthesis (Wynne-Davies and Scott., 1979), delay in bone healing after fracture (Kujala et al., 1992), just mentioning some studies in a orthopedics context. The hypothesis in patients suffering from generalized tendinopathy (that may include rotator cuff pathology, epicondylopathy, carpal tunnel syndrome, triggering of the long finger flexor tendons and extensor tendon pathology such as de Quervain's disease) of a "mesenchymal syndrome", theorizing about a possible genetic component that could cause an abnormal formation of collagen was advanced by Nirshil (Nirshl, 1969). He was comforted in his theory by the fact that in this group, normal routine rheumatologic tests were normal. In general tendinopathy context, Achilles tendon has a particularly important aspect. Achilles tendinopathy and ruptures are increasing among the non-sporting population as well (Young and Maffulli., 2007). In this regard, several etiological hypotheses were formulated (Knörzer et al., 1986; Joza et al., 1989; Selvanetti et al., 1997; Maffulli, 1999; Vanek et al., 2003) but in any case, the etiology remains multifactorial (Bestwick and Maffulli, 2000; Wilson and Goodship, 1994).

From an anatomical point of view, as in any case, it is important to remember how the Achilles tendon received the blood supply. The tendon vascularity comes from two arteries which run longitudinally to the tendon belly. A part of its blood supply comes from vessels running in the paratenon that are mainly derived from the posterior tibial artery. An additional supply in the proximal part of the tendon is furnished by the muscle bellies that continues into the tendon via the endotenon, (in any case this contribution is not significant). Finally, the distal region receives vessels from an arterial periosteal plexus on the posterior aspect of the calcaneus. The Achilles tendon has, in its downward course, a kind of anatomical twist starting above the point at which is the fusion with the solearis tendon portion. This twist is much more evident as less is important the solearis fusion (Jozsa e Kannus, 1997). This twist causes the emergence of a stress area resulting in a lesser blood flow, displaced about 2-6 centimeters above the tendon heel insertion. For this reason, this area is the site most commonly encountered for pathological risk.

From a structural point of view, the Achilles tendon shows a tenocytes and tenoblasts percentage equal approximately to 90-95% of its cellular elements. Collagen and elastin are present at levels of about 70 and 2% respectively of the dry weight of the tendon structure and form the most part of the extracellular matrix. The collagen production in the tendon can be affected by many factors, such as the inheritance, the diet, the nerve supply, besides genetic and hormonal factors (Viidik., 1973). Corticosteroids inhibit the new collagen growth while insulin, estrogen and testosterone favor it (O'Brien, 2005). Even the mechanical stimulus related to physical exercise promotes the new collagen synthesis, the increase in the myofibrils number and size and the metabolic enzymes concentration. This will result in increasing the tendon tensile strength (O'Brien, 2005). The Achilles tendon has a high capacity to withstand the tensional forces created by the movements. In vivo peak force of the Achilles tendon has been measured at more than 2.200 Newtons (Fukashiro et al., 1995), namely in the order of 50-100 N/mm (Waggett et al., 1998). However, Achilles tendon transmits forces that are approximately seven times the subject body weight during activity such as running, this represents a huge increase on the forces that normally act during standing which are about half the body weight(Ker et al., 1987). When the Achilles tendon is subjected to tensile stress its wavy configuration disappears and its collagen fibers respond in linear manner to increasing load and a strain level greater than 8% leads to macroscopic rupture due to tensile failure of the tendon collagen fibers (O'Brien, 1992)

Collagen type most represented is the type I, with a rate of approximately 95% (Kastelic et al., 1978; Maffulli and Benazzo, 2000). Type I collagen fibrils are grouped into fibers, fiber bundles, and fascicles, so that the Achilles tendon is a very similar to a multistranded cable. However, Achilles tendons which have undergone a complete rupture, show an increase of type III and type V collagen which are known to be less resistant against tensile stress (Coombs et al., 1980; Wren et al., 2000; Koob and Vogel, 1987; Benjamin and Ralphs, 1998). In fact, the type III collagen is mainly present in the tendon during the healing process (Jósza e Kannus, 1997; Myerson and McGarvey, 1999) while type V collagen increases with the tendon aging process and is associated with a decrease in diameter of tendon fibers as well with a decrease in its mechanical properties (Dressler et al., 2002; Goncalves-Neto et al., 2002). In fact, some studies have shown that the tenocytes, following a damaging and / or degenerative event, show an increase in type III and V collagen production that perturb the tendon tissue architecture decreasing its stress resistance (Waterston e coll., 1997). Also other Authors underline that an important proportion of type I collagen increases the strength of the tendon structure (Butler e coll., 1978) and that the minor structural strength of type III and V collagen compared with type I collagen is attributable to the fact that the first two types (III and V) have fewer crosslink than the second one (I) (Józsa e coll., 1990). In addition, some studies indicate an inverse correlation between the type III collagen reactivity and diameter, and thus the structural strength, of tendon fibers (Birk e Maine, 1997). So, a repeated micro-injuries history to the Achilles tendon level may lead to the formation of a hypertrophic tendon tissue which is biologically weaker and which also tends to replace the normal tissue.

In fact, during the normal physiological activity, some microscopic breaks occur in the tendon substance. They are continually remodeled by the formation of new collagen. Obviously, this destruction-remodeling process is particularly emphasized in some sports activities, as for example the run, that strongly stresses the tendon structure (Kirkendall, 1997; Selvanetti et al., 1997). Subjects belonging to blood group 0 shows a N-acetylgalactosamine transferase activity much higher than in subjects in A and B group (Kujala e coll., 1992). This increased N-acetylgalactosamine transferase activity would be result in an increase in type III collagen production within the tendon.

Since the type III collagen shows less resistance against mechanical stress compared to type I collagen (Waterston e Maffulli, 1997), its abnormal proliferation may expose to tendinopathy, which could end in tendon spontaneous rupture (Joza et al., 1989; Maffulli, 1999; Maffulli et al., 2000). Is also interesting to note that recently a type III collagen abnormal proliferation and a decreasing in type I collagen are always present in the Achilles tendon calcific insertional tendinopathy (Maffulli et al., 2010). Interesting to note that, since the ABO gene encodes for transferases, some studies have suggested that the different enzymes produced by the ABO gene, could determine not only the glycoprotein antigens structure determination on the red blood cells, but also some types of glycoproteins found within the ground tendons substance (Jozsa et al., 1989). Other studies have proposed that other genes, closely linked to the ABO gene on the tip of the long arm of chromosome 9q32-q34, which encode for components of the extracellular matrix, are more likely associated with Achilles tendon pathology (.Kannus and Natri, 1997; Kujala et al., 1992).

Two of these genes, tenascin-C gene and COL5A1, encode for structural components of tendons (Mokone et al., 2005). The COL5A1 gene encodes for the pro alpha1 (V) collagen chain, found in most of the isoforms of type V collagen (Birk, 2001; Silver et al., 2003).

In literature, we can find other examples concerning other pathologies, such as the nail-patella syndrome, where the LMX1B gene, is closely linked to the ABO gene, encoded for a protein responsible for the pathology (Bongers et al. 2002).

However, as already suggested by other Authors (Adam and Maffulli, 2007), it is highly unlikely that a single gene, or a group of genes, are exclusively associated with the development of the symptoms of Achilles tendon injury. In fact, it's more probable that this condition is polygenic, and other genes that encode for important structural components of tendons are also associated with Achilles tendon injury.

In any case, the above could explain the high incidence of the Achilles tendon spontaneous ruptures found by some Authors in individuals belonging to blood group 0 than in A and B group (Joza e al., 1989; Maffulli, 1999). Furthermore, it is interesting to underline that the type III and V collagen high percentage would may explain the occurrence of a spontaneous rupture in tendons that does not show previous degenerative processes.

In our subjects, the group 0 most found frequency (66.6% $p<0.005$) confirms the hypothesis of an increased susceptibility of individuals belonging to this group in developing tendinopathy at Achilles tendon level and would agree with previous results findings by others Authors (Joza e al., 1989; Maffulli, 1999). Obviously, the limited sample that we considered in our study does not allow us to affirm with certainty this hypothesis which should be confirmed by further studies to be carried out on a larger population. For this reason the results of our study must be interpreted with the greatest attention taking into account this limitation.

In any case, this finding seems particularly interesting in a sporting context, especially concerning its possible use as a preventive measure. In fact, our study may suggest the importance for athletes belonging to 0 group, that practice a sporting activity, such as football, athletics, jogging, running, and/or at least all the other sporting activities which strongly encourage stress to the Achilles tendon, to carry out a regular preventive program based primarily on increasing the Achilles tendon eccentric strength (Allison and Purdam, 2009; Gärdin et al., 2009).

In conclusion, during a sporting activity there is a high incidence of tendon injuries, however, the exact etiology of this condition is not yet fully understood. Some studies, to which our study is a part of, suggest that the genetic component can play an important role; so given the interest and the importance of these problems, we hope that in the future, others studies will further clarify and deepen this exciting topic.

10. Appendix A

Soft tissue diagnostic ultrasound examination of the Achilles tendon

Right Achilles tendon:

Tendon:

- Shape:

- Angular: __
- Fusiform: __
- Margin:
  - Sharply defined __
  - Poorly defined __
- Contour:
  - Smooth __
  - Nodular __
  - Tapered __
- Max. diameter:
  - AP: _____ mm
  - TRV: _____ mm
- Internal architecture
  - Organised __
  - Central hypoechoic foci (med/lat/ant/post)__
  - Disrupted fibres (mild/mod/severe) __
  - Haematoma __
  - Calcification __
  - Acoustic shadowing __
- Power Doppler vascularity
  - Absent __
  - Present __
  - Prominent __

Paratenon

- Fluid:
  - Absent __
  - Present
    - Site _____
    - Amount _____
- Soft tissue swelling
  - Absent __
  - Present __
- Power Doppler Vascularity
  - Absent __
  - Present __
  - Increased __
- Retrocalcaneal Bursa
  - Normal __
  - Fluid filled __
- Kager's fat
  - Normal __
  - Hyperechogenic __

Myotendinous junction

- Normal __

- Tear __

Calcaneus

- Normal __
- Abnormal __

Left Achilles tendon:

Tendon:

- Shape:
  - Angular: __
  - Fusiform: __
- Margin:
  - Sharply defined __
  - Poorly defined __
- Contour:
  - Smooth __
  - Nodular __
  - Tapered __
- Max. diameter:
  - AP: _____ mm
  - TRV: _____ mm
- Internal architecture
  - Organised __
  - Central hypoechoic foci (med/lat/ant/post)__
  - Disrupted fibres (mild/mod/severe) __
  - Haematoma __
  - Calcification __
  - Acoustic shadowing __
- Power Doppler vascularity
  - Absent __
  - Present __
  - Prominent __

Paratenon

- Fluid:
  - Absent __
  - Present
    - Site _____
    - Amount _____
- Soft tissue swelling
  - Absent __
  - Present __
- Power Doppler Vascularity
  - Absent __

- Present __
- Increased __
- Retrocalcaneal Bursa
  - Normal __
  - Fluid filled __
- Kager's fat
  - Normal __
  - Hyperechogenic __

Myotendinous junction

- Normal __
- Tear __

Calcaneus

- Normal __
- Abnormal __

11. References

Adam A., Maffulli N. *Genes and Achilles tendon. In: The Achilles Tendon.* Nicola Maffulli and Louis C. Almekinders (Eds). Springer-Verlag London Limited 2007.

Aird I., Bentall HH., Fraser-Robert JA. Statistical analysis. A relationship between cancer of stomach and ABO blood groups. Br Med J. 2: 799-801, 1953.

Ajis A., Maffulli N. Genes and the Achilles Tendon. In: Achilles tendon. Mafulli N and Almekinders LC (Ed). Springer-Verlag London Limited 2007

Ajis A., Maffulli N., Alfredson H., Almekinders L. Tendinopaty of the main body of the Achilles tendon. In: Tendon injuries Maffulli N., Renström P., Leadbetter WB (Ed). Springer-Verlag London Limited 2005

Alison V September, Martin P Schwellnus, Malcolm Collins. Tendon and ligament injuries: the genetic component Br J Sports Med 2007;41:241–246. doi: 10.1136/bjsm.2006.033035.

Allison GT, Purdam C. Eccentric loading for Achilles tendinopathy--strengthening or stretching? Br J Sports Med. 2009 Apr;43(4):276-9.

Arner O, Lindholm A. (1959) Histologic changes in subcutaneous rupture of the Achilles tendon. Acta Chir Scand. 116:484–490.

Barfred T. (1971) Experimental rupture of the Achilles tendon. Acta Orthop Scand. 42:528–543.

Benjamin M, Ralphs JR. (1998) Fibrocartilage in tendonsand ligaments—an adaptation to compressive load. J Anat.193:481–494.

Beretta M, Mazzetti P, Mamolini E, Gavina R, Barale R, Vullo C, Ravani A, Franze A, Sapigni T, Soracco E. Genetic structure of the human population in the Po delta. Am J Hum Genet. 1989 Jul;45(1):49-62

Bestwick CS, Maffulli N. Reactive oxygen species and tendon problems: review and hypothesis. Sports Med Arthroscopy Rev 2000; 8:6–16.

Birk DE. Type V collagen: Heterotypic type I/V collagen interactions in the regulation of fi bril assembly. Micron 2001 Apr; 32(3):223–237.

Birk DE., Mayne R. Localization of collagen types I, III, and V during tendon development: Changes in collagen types I and III are correlated with changes in fibril diameter. Eur L Cell Biol. 1997; 72: 352-361.

Bongers EM, Gubler MC, Knoers NV. Nail-patella syndrome: Overview on clinical and molecular findings. Pediatr Nephrol 2002 Sep; 17(9):703–712.

Butler DL, Grood ES, Noyes FR, Zernicke RF. (1978) Biomechanics of ligaments and tendons. Exerc Sports Sci Rev.6:125–182.

Cetti R, Christensen SE. (1983) Surgical treatment under local anesthesia of Achilles tendon rupture. Clin Orthop Rel Res. (173):204–208.

Clain MR., Baxter DE. Achilles tendinitis. Foot and Ankle 1992; 13(8):482–487

Clement DB., Taunton JE., Smart GW. Achilles tendinitis and peritendinitis: Etiology and treatment. Am J Sports Med 1984; 12(3):179–184

Collins M., Dijkstra P., Raleigh S., Ribbans B. Colllins M., Dijkstra P., Raleigh S., Ribbans B. Genetic Basis of Soft Tissue Injuries in Elite Athletes - A Prospective Cohort Study (ongoing study, 2010)

Coombs RRH, Klenerman L, Narcisi P, Nichols A, Pope FM. (1980) Collagen typing in Achilles tendon rupture.J Bone Joint Surg. 62-B(2):258.

Corps AN, Curry VA, Harrall RL, Dutt D, Hazleman BL, Riley GP. Ciprofloxacin reduces the stimulation of prostaglandin E(2) output by interleukin-1beta in human tendon-derived cells. Rheumatology 2003; 42(11):1306–1310.

Davidsson L, Salo M. (1969) Pathogenesis of subcutaneous Achilles tendon ruptures. Acta Chir Scand. 135:209–212.

Dodds WN, Burry HC. The relationship between Achilles tendon rupture and serum uric acid level. Injury. 1984 Sep;16(2):94-5

Dressler MR, Butler DL, Wenstrup R, Awad HA, Smith F, Boivin GP. A potential mechanism for agerelated declines in patellar tendon biomechanics. J Orthop Res 2002 Nov; 20(6):1315–1322.

Eid M. Acute haematogenous osteomyelitis and ABO blood groups and secretor status. Arch Orthop Trauma Surg. 104: 106-108, 1985.

Filippucci E., Farina A., Bartolucci F.,. Spallacci C., Busilacchi P.,. Grassi W. Fluoroquinolone-induced bilateral rupture of the Achilles tendon: clinical and sonographic findings. Reumatismo, 2003; 55(4):267-269.

Fisher P. Role of steroids in tendon rupture or disintegration known for decades. Arch Intern Med 2004; 164:678.

Fox JM, Blazina ME, Jobe FW, Kerlan RK, Carter VS, Shields CL Jr, Carlson GJ. (1975) Degeneration and rupture of the Achilles tendon. Clin Orthop Rel Res. (107):221–224.

Fukashiro S, Komi PV, Jarvinen M, Miyashita M. In vivo Achilles tendon loading during jumping in humans. Eur J Appl Physiol Occup Physiol 1995; 71(5):453–458.

Gärdin A, Movin T, Svensson L, Shalabi A. The long-term clinical and MRI results following eccentric calf muscle training in chronic Achilles tendinosis. Skeletal Radiol. 2010 May;39(5):435-42.

Giaccone P, Procaccianti S, Scalici E, Sammarco M. Distribution of blood groups in the population of Palermo and its province. Acta Med Leg Soc (Liege). 1982;32:543-8.

Goncalves-Neto J, Witzel SS, Teodoro WR, Carvalho-Junior AE, Fernandes TD, Yoshinari HH. Changes in collagen matrix composition in human posterior tibial tendon dysfunction. Joint BoneSpine 2002 Mar; 69(2):189-194.

Gottschalk AW, Andrish JT. Epidemiology of sports injury in pediatric athletes. Sports Med Arthrosc. 2011 Mar;19(1):2-6.

Hess GP, Capiello WL, Poole RM, Hunter SC. (1989) Prevention and treatment of overuse tendon injuries. SportsMed. 8:371-384.

Hestin D, Mainard D, Pere P, Bellou A, Renoult E, Cao Huu T, Chanliau J, Kessler M. Spontaneous bilateral rupture of the Achilles tendons in a renal transplant recipient. Nephron. 1993; 65(3)491-492.

Huston KA. Achilles tendinitis and tendon ruptures due to fluoroquinolone antibiotics. N Engl J Med 1994; 331: 748.

James SL., Bates BT., Osternig LR. Injuries to runners. Am J Sports Med 1978; 6(2):40-50.

Järvinen M, Jozsa L, Kannus P, Jarvinen TL, Kvist M, Leadbetter W. (1997) Histopathological findings in chronic tendon disorders. Scand J Med Sci Sports. 7(2):86-95.

Järvinen TAH., Kannus P, Józsa L., Paavola M., Järvinen TLN., Järvinen M. Achilles tendon injuries. Curr Opin Rheumatol 2001; 13(2):150-155.

Jósza L, Kannus P. Human Tendons—Anatomy, Physiology and Pathology. Champaign, IL: Human Kinetics, 1997.

Józsa L, Kannus P, Balint JB, Reffy A. Threedimensional ultrastructure of human tendons. Acta Anat. 1991; 142(4):306-312.

Józsa L, Kannus P. Histopathological findings in spontaneous tendon ruptures. Scand J Med Sci Sports. 1997; 7(2):113-118.

Józsa L, Reffy A, Kannus P, Demel S, Elek E. Pathological alterations in human tendons. Arch Orthop TraumaSurg. 1990; 110(1):15-21.

Józsa L., Balint JB., Kannus P., Reffy A., Barzo M. Distrubution of blood groups in patients with tendon rupture. An analysis of 832 cases. J Bone Joint Surg. 1989; 71B: 272-274.

Józsa L., Kannus P. Human Tendons: Anatomy, Physiology, and Pathology. Champaign, IL: Human Kinetics, 1997.

Kannus P, Józsa L. (1991) Histopathological changes preceding spontaneous rupture of a tendon: a controlled study of 891 patients. J Bone Joint Surg. (Am) 73(10): 1507-1525.

Kannus P, Natri A. Etiology and pathophysiology of tendon ruptures in sports. Scand J Med Sci Sports 1997 Apr; 7(2):107-112.

Kannus P. Etiology and pathophysiology of chronic tendon disorders in sports. Scand J Sports Med 1997; 7(2):78-85.

Kastelic J, Galeski A, Baer E. The multi-compositestructure of tendon. Connect Tissue Res. 1978;6:11-23.

Kaufman KR., Brodine SK., Shaffer RA., Johnson CW., Cullison TR. The effect of foot structure and range of motion on musculoskeletal overuse injuries. Am J Sports Med 1999; 27:585-593.

Kearney R, Costa ML. Insertional Achilles tendinopathy management: a systematic review. Foot Ankle Int. 2010 Aug;31(8):689-94

Ker RF, Bennett MB, Bibby SR, Kester RC, Alexander RM. The spring in the arch of the human foot. Nature 1987; 325:147-149.

Kirkendall DT. Function and biomechanics of tendons. Scand J Med Sci Sports. 1997; 7(2):62–66.

Knörzer E, Folkhard W, Geercken W, Boschert C, Koch MH, Hilbert B, Krahl H, Mosler E, Nemetschek-Gansler H, Nemetschek T. New aspects of the aetiology of tendon rupture: An analysis of time-resolved dynamic mechanical measurements using synchotron radiation. Arch Orthop Trauma Surg. 1986; 105:113–120.

Koob TJ,Vogel KG. Proteoglycan synthesis in organcultures from different regions of bovine tendon subjectedto different mechanical forces. Biochem J.1987; 246:589–598.

Kujala UM, Jarvinen M, Natri A, Lehto M, Nelimarkka O, Hurme M, Virta L, Finne J. ABO bloodgroups and musculoskeletal injuries. Injury 1992; 23(2):131–133.

Kvist M. Achilles tendon injuries in athletes. Sports Med 1994; 18:173–201.

Kvist M. Achilles tendon injuries in athletes. Ann Chir Gynaecol 1991; 80(2):188–201.

Linden Van Der P., Sturkenboom M., Herings R., Leufkens H., Rowlands S., Stricker B. Increased risk of Achilles tendon rupture with quinolone antibacterial use, especially in elderly patients taking oral corticosteroids. Arch Intern Med 2003; 163:1801–1807.

Lourie JA. Is there an association between ABO blood group antigens and primary osteoarthrosis of the hip? Ann Hum Biol. 1983; 10:381-383.

Maffulli N, Benazzo F. Basic Science of tendons. Sports. Med Arthroscopy Rev. 2000; 8:(1)1–5.

Maffulli N, Ewen SW, Waterston SW, Reaper J, Barrass V. Tenocytes from ruptured and tendinopathic achilles tendons produce greater quantities of type III collagen than tenocytes from normal Achilles tendons: An in vitro model of human tendon healing. Am J Sports Med 2000; 28: 499–505.

Maffulli N, Kader D. Tendinopathy of tendo Achilles. J Bone Joint Surg Br 2002; 84:1–8.

Maffulli N, Longo UG, Maffulli GD, Rabitti C, Khanna A, Denaro V. Marked pathological changes proximal and distal to the site of rupture in acute Achilles tendon ruptures. Knee Surg Sports Traumatol Arthrosc. 2010 Jun 19. [Epub ahead of print]

Maffulli N. Rupture of the Achilles tendon. J Bone Joint Surg. (Am) 1999; 81(7):1019–1036.

Mahieu NN, Witvrouw E, Stevens V, Van Tiggelen D, Roget P. Intrinsic risk factors for the development of Achilles tendon overuse injury: A prospective study. Am J Sports Med 2006; 34(2):226–235.

Mancia G, Volpe R, Boros S, Ilardi M, Giannattasio C. Cardiovascular risk profile and blood pressure control in Italian hypertensive patients under specialist care. J Hypertens. 2004 Jan;22(1):51-7.

Mathiak G., Wening JV., Mathiak M., Neville LF., Jungbluth K. Serum cholesterol is elevated in patients with Achilles tendon ruptures. Arch Orthop Trauma Surg 1999; 119:280–284.

Mazzone MF, McCue T. Common conditions of the Achilles tendon. Am Fam Physician 2002;65:1805–10.

Min W, Ding BC, Sheskier S. Technical tip: use of the Kerrison rongeur through a single-incision exposure for resection of Haglund's deformity. Foot Ankle Int. 2010 Nov;31(11):1028-31

Moira O'Brien. Anatomy of tendons. In: Maffulli N., Renström P., Leadbetter WP. (Editors). Tendon Injuries.Basic Science and Clinical Medicine. Springer-Verlag London Limited 2005. pp: 11-12.

Mokone GG, Gajjar M, September AV, Schwellnus MP, Greenberg J, Noakes TD, Collins M. The guanine-thymine dinucleotide repeat polymorphism within the tenascin-C gene is associated with Achilles tendon injuries. Am J Sports Med 2005 Jul; 33(7):1016–1021.

Moller A, Astron M, Westlin N. Increasing incidence of Achilles tendon rupture. Acta Orthop Scand. 1996; 67(5):479–481.

Myerson MS, McGarvey W. (1999) Disorders of the Achilles tendon insertion and Achilles tendinitis. InstrCourse Lect. 48:211–218.

Newnham D, Douglas J, Legge J, Friend J. Achilles tendon rupture: An underrated complication of corticosteroid treatment. Thorax 1991; 46:853–854.

Nirschl RP. Mesenchymal syndrome. Virginia Med Mon. 1969; 96:659.

O'Brien M. Functional anatomy and physiology of tendons. Clin Sports Med 1992; 11:505–520

Ozgurtas T., Yildiz C., Serdar M., Atesalp S., Kutluay T. Is high concentration of serum lipids a risk factor for Achilles tendon rupture? Clin Chim Acta 2003; 331:25–28.

Palmieri L, Trojani M, Vanuzzo D, Panico S, Pilotto L, Dima F, Noce CL, Uguccioni M, Pede S, Giampaoli S. Distribution of the global cardiovascular risk in the Italian population: results from the cardiovascular epidemiologic observatory. Ital Heart J Suppl. 2005 May;6(5):279-84

Piazza A, Cappello N, Olivetti E, Rendine S. A genetic history of Italy. Ann Hum Genet. 1988 Jul;52(Pt 3):203-13

Porcella P, Vona G. Distribution of the ABO system and Rh factor in Sardinia. Anthropol Anz. 1987 Dec;45(4):309-21

Rees JD, Wilson AM, Wolman RL. Current concepts in the management of tendon disorders. Rheumatology. 2006;45:508–21.

Renwick J. H. and Lawler S. D. (1955) Genetical linkage between the ABO and nail-patella loci. Am. J. Hum. Genet. 19, 312.

Ribard P, Audiso F, Kahn MF.Seven Achilles tendonitis cases including 3 complicated by rupture during fluoroquinolone therapy. J Rheumatol 1992; 19(9):1479–1481

Rickards O, Scano G, Martinez-Labarga C, Taraborelli T, Gruppioni G, De Stefano GF. Genetic history of the population of Puglia (southern Italy). Gene Geogr. 1995 Apr;9(1):25-40

Roggi C, Minoia C, Silva S, Ronchi A, Gatti A, Maccarini L. Distribution of blood lead level in a general population. Ann Ig. 1995 Sep-Oct;7(5):359-67.

Royer RJ, Pierfitte C, Netter P. Features of tendon disorders with fluoroquinolones. Therapie 1994; 49:75–76.

Ryan M, Grau S, Krauss I, Maiwald C, Taunton J, Horstmann T. Kinematic analysis of runners with achilles mid-portion tendinopathy. Foot Ankle Int. 2009 Dec; 30(12):1190-1997.

Schepsis AA, Jones H, Haas AL. Achilles tendon disorders in athletes. Am.J Sports Med 2002;30:287-305.

Schwellnus MP, Derman EW, Noakes TD. Aetiology of skeletal muscle 'cramps' during exercise: a novel hypothesis. J Sports Sci. 1997 Jun;15(3):277-85.

Selvanetti A, Cipolla M, Puddu G. Overuse tendon injuries: basic science and classification. Op Tech Sports Med. 1997; 5(3):110–117.

Silver FH, Freeman JW, Seehra GP. Collagen self-assembly and the development of tendon mechanical properties. J Biomech 2003 Oct; 36(10):1529–1553.

Speed CA. Corticosteroid injections in tendon lesions. BMJ 2001; 323:382–386.

Szarfman A, Chen M, Blum MD, Pierfitte C, Gillet P,Royer RJ. More on fluoroquinolone antibiotics and tendon rupture. N Engl J Med 1995; 332: 193.

Unverferth L, Olix M. The effect of local steroid injections on tendon. In: Proceedings of the American Academy of Orthopaedic Surgeons. J Bone Joint Surg Am 1973; 55:1315.

Vanek D, Saxena A, Boggs JM. Fluoroquinolone therapy and Achilles tendon rupture. J Am Podiatr Med Assoc. 2003; 93:333–335.

Vanek D, Saxena A, Boggs JM. Fluoroquinolone therapy and Achilles tendon rupture. J Am Podiatr Med Assoc. 2003; 93:333–335.

Viidik A. Functional properties of collagenous tissues. Rev Connect Tissue Res. 1973; 6:127–215.

Vona G, Salis M, Bitti P, Succa V. Blood groups of the Sardinian population (Italy). Anthropol Anz. 1994 Dec;52(4):297-304.

Waggett AD, Ralphs JR, Kwan AP, Woodnutt D, Benjamin M. Characterization of collagens and proteoglycans at the insertion of the human Achilles tendon. Matrix Biol 1998; 16:457–470.

Waterston SW, Maffulli N, Ewen SW. Subcutaneous rupture of the Achilles tendon: basic science and some aspects of clinical practice. Br J Sports Med. 1997; 31(4):285–298.

Waterston SW. Histochemistry and biochemistry of Achilles tendon ruptures. University of Aberdeen (Ed). 1–58, 1997.

Williams JG. (1986) Achilles tendon lesions in sport. SportsMed. 3(2):114–135.

Wilson AM, Goodship AE. Exercise-induced hyperthermia as a possible mechanism for tendon degeneration. J Biomech 1994; 27(7):899–905.

Wren TAL, Beaupre GS, Carter DR. Mechanobiology of tendon adaptation to compressive loadingthrough fibrocartilaginous metaplasia. J Rehabil Res Dev.2000; 37:135–143.

Wyndow N, Cowan SM, Wrigley TV, Crossley KM. Neuromotor control of the lower limb in Achilles tendinopathy: implications for foot orthotic therapy. Sports Med. 2010 Sep 1;40(9):715-2

Wynne-Davies R. and Scott J. H. S. Inheritance and spondylolisthesis. J Borte Joint Surg. 1979; 61B, 301.

Young SJ., Maffulli N. Etiology and epidemiology of Achilles tendon problem. In: Maffulli N., Almekinders LC (Editors). The Achilles Tendon. Springer-Verlag London Limited, 2007.

7

Surgical Treatment of the Neglected Achilles Tendon Rupture

Jake Lee and John M. Schuberth
Kaiser Foundation Hospital, San Francisco, CA
USA

1. Introduction

The true frequency of acute Achilles tendon rupture is unknown but historically it was regarded as a rare injury comprising less than 0.2% of the general population (Cetti et al., 1993; Nillius et al., 1976). However, in the past decade the incidence of Achilles tendon rupture has increased (Maffuli et al., 1999). At the present time, Achilles tendon ruptures are the most common tendon rupture of the lower extremity and may account for up to 40% of all operated tendon ruptures (Habusta, 1995; Jozsa et al., 1989). The increase in frequency is thought to be due to an increased interest and participation in recreational sports by middle-aged and older patients and also to better reporting (Coughlin et al, 2007).

In many patients the initial symptoms after an Achilles tendon rupture diminish quickly. In a study of 57 patients with acute Achilles rupture, 19 of them reported to be painless (Christensen, 1953). Patients with Achilles tendon ruptures frequently are unable to stand on the toes of the involved side, however, active plantarflexion maybe intact due to partial ruptures, recruitment of plantar flexors, and an intact plantaris muscle. The lack of pain and no obvious loss of plantarflexion can be misleading and up to 20-25% of cases the diagnosis is missed initially (Maffuli, 1996; Arner & Lindholm, 1959; Nillius et al., 1976). The failure to establish the diagnosis at the initial presentation is the most common reason for delayed treatment.

There are many terms used to describe this condition and treatment, including neglected or chronic rupture, late or old repair, and delayed reconstruction (Abraham & Pankovich, 1975; Ozaki et al., 1989; Porter et al., 1997). There is no consensus regarding the specific time in which an acute becomes a neglected rupture although 4 weeks may be the most widely accepted interval (Leppilahti & Orava, 1998; Porter et al., 1997). Contraction of the triceps surae complex has been observed 3 to 4 days post-injury (Bosworth, 1956). Regardless of the lack of a chronological definition, neglected ruptures are characterized by the difficulty of achieving an end-to-end apposition of the tendon ends with plantarflexion of the foot during surgical reconstruction.

Neglected ruptures can heal without surgery as abundant scar tissue has been shown to form in the rupture interval (Barnes & Hardy, 1986). However, due to the contracture of the triceps surae complex, the resulting functional length of the muscle-tendon unit may be too long even with re-establishment of the continuity of the muscle tendon complex through scar tissue formation. This leads to comprised plantarflexion power, reducing ankle stability and an impaired gait pattern.

1.1 Clinical evaluation

A palpable gap is rarely felt on physical examinations at the previous rupture site due to scar tissue formation. However with careful digital palpation or direct visual inspection, the site of the neglected rupture can often be determined due to a change in the consistency of the tissue and a change in contour of the posterior leg **[Figure 1]**. The additional findings on clinical examination will depend on the functional length of the healed tendon. Patients will display increased dorsiflexion of the ankle joint and decreased plantarflexion power compared to the contralateral limb. Patients often report that they are easily fatigued with sports. It is highly unlikely that they are able to perform a single limb heel rise. During gait there is delayed heel-off and a shortened stride. Magnetic Resonance Imaging (MRI) is a useful tool in confirming the clinical diagnosis but more so for assessing the amount of functional defect within the Achilles tendon for preoperative planning **[Figure 2]**.

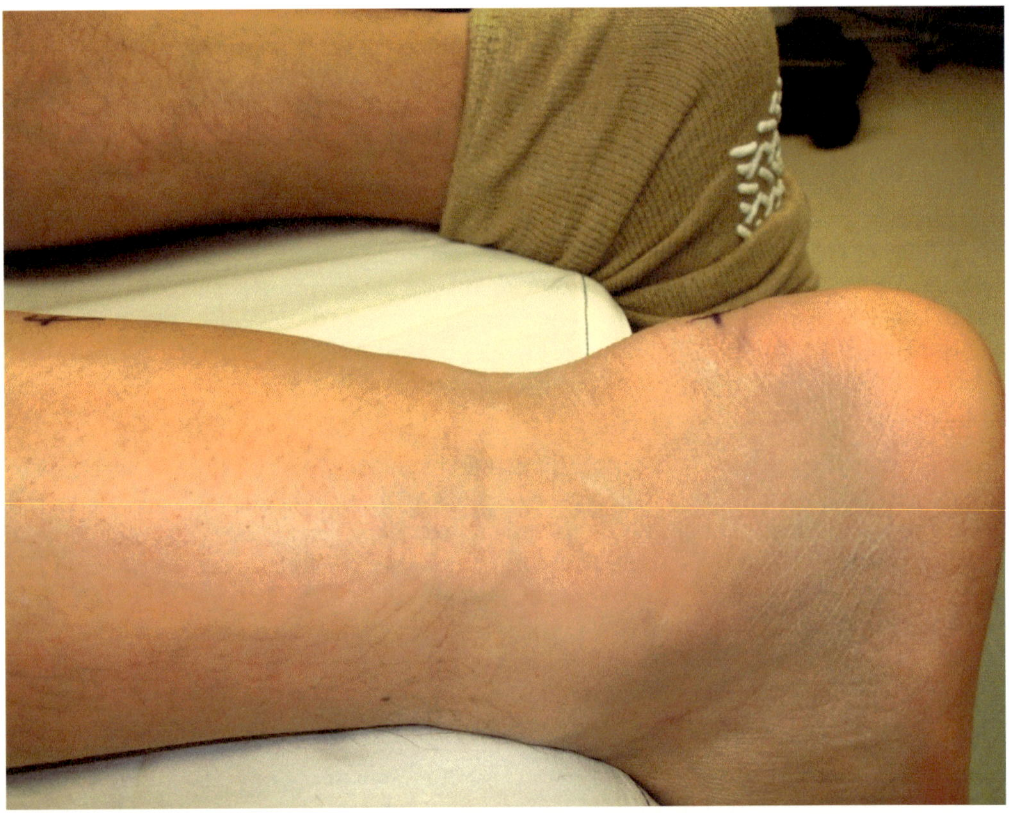

Fig. 1. Delayed presentation with clinically evident defect in the Achilles tendon

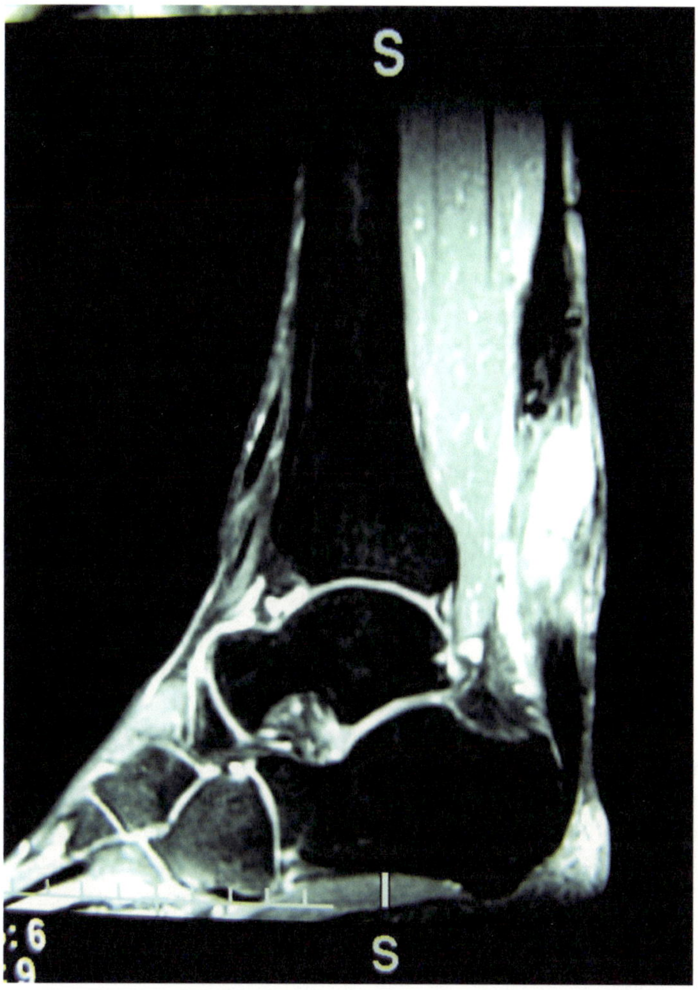

Fig. 2. Magnetic Resonance Imaging demonstrating a large defect in a patient with a neglected Achilles tendon rupture

2. Conservative treatment

The best functional outcomes are achieved through surgical reconstruction but non-surgical treatment may be preferable for patients with poor skin condition, history of smoking, soft tissue complications from previous surgery, and poorly controlled long-standing diabetes mellitus. Conservative treatment could be as simple as lace up ankle brace or custom made leather ankle brace (i.e. - Arizona brace). In patients with severe Achilles dysfunction, an Ankle-Foot-Orthosis (AFO) can be considered. Any bracing method can be coupled with physical therapy to strengthen the gastrocnemius and recruitment of the entire deep posterior compartment muscles.

The use of immobilization for treatment of neglected ruptures is suspect, but may be more useful prior to the maturation of the interposed scar in the post-injury period. If conservative treatment is chosen, it is important to realize that the immobilization period will be much longer. Serial casting with reduction of the equinus position of the foot at each visit may allow for consolidation and re-establishment of functional continuity. However each respective casting stage will be extended compared to non-operative treatment of an acute rupture. Ultrasound can offer some assistance in assessing the extent of fibrous tissue in the gap. It can serve as a prognostic indicator as well as a tool in guiding how much equinus is needed for tendon apposition. Initial immobilization in a long leg cast with the knee at 25 degrees and the appropriate level of equinus of the ankle has been proposed. This initial cast is kept for 4 weeks. Subsequent serial casting is done every 3 weeks with successive reduced equinus over the span of 7-10 weeks or once the tendon continuity is ensured clinically. This is followed by conversion to a short leg cast with gradual serial reduction of any residual equinus. (Schuberth, 1996)

3. Surgical treatment

Many surgical techniques have been described for the management of neglected Achilles ruptures. The primary goal of any surgical treatment is to restore the function and strength of the gastrocnemius-soleus complex by recreating the optimal length-tension relationship. End-to-end repair is ideal if the gap between tendon ends allow direct apposition after resection of the interposed scar tissue. This will allow for maximum isokinetic strength of Achilles because re-establishment of the pre-injury tendon length can only be achieved. It is generally accepted that approximately 1-2 cm gap will allow end-to-end repair (Myerson, 2010) **[Figure 3]**. However, primary repair is still an uncommon form of treatment for most chronic ruptures because of the potential for shortening and contracture of the gastrocnemius-soleus muscle-tendon unit. (Bosworth, 1956). Excision of scar tissue from neglected rupture often results in a sizable gap requiring other modalities to bridge the defect. If the gap exceeds 1-2 cm and primary repair is still deemed feasible, proximal lengthening of the gastro-soleal complex may be utilized to achieve mobilization of the proximal tendon end to facilitate primary repair. These techniques were developed primarily because of the dissatisfaction with the fascial turn down techniques (Abraham & Pankovich, 1975). Porter et al. reported on end-to-end primary repair without augmentation of chronic ruptures (greater than or equal to 4 weeks and less than equal to 12 weeks from injury) in 11 patients. Proximal gastro-soleal complex release was performed with imbrication of the fibrous scar tissue without excision of local tissue. Primary repair of the tendon ends was then performed. In an average follow up of 3.5 years no re-ruptures were observed and patients were able to return to pre-injury level of activities in an average of 5.8 months. Total ankle range of motion (ROM) was comparable to the uninjured side. The loss of plantarflexion power and pain scale ratings were similar to the patients surgically treated after an acute rupture repair performed by the same surgeon (Porter et al., 1997).

Gastrocnemius slide lengthening techniques have also been utilized to achieve end-to-end anastomosis (Barnes and Hardy, 1987) (Abraham & Pankovich, 1975). In this technique, an inverted V incision is made into the aponeurosis then with traction on the distal tendon it is repaired in a Y fashion. The arms of the V incision should at least one and a half times the length of the defect to allow suturing in a Y shape. The size of defects after excision of scar tissue ranged from 5cm to 6cm with the ankle in plantarflexion in their series and in 3 out 4 patients in their study full plantarflexion strength was restored (Abraham & Pankovich,

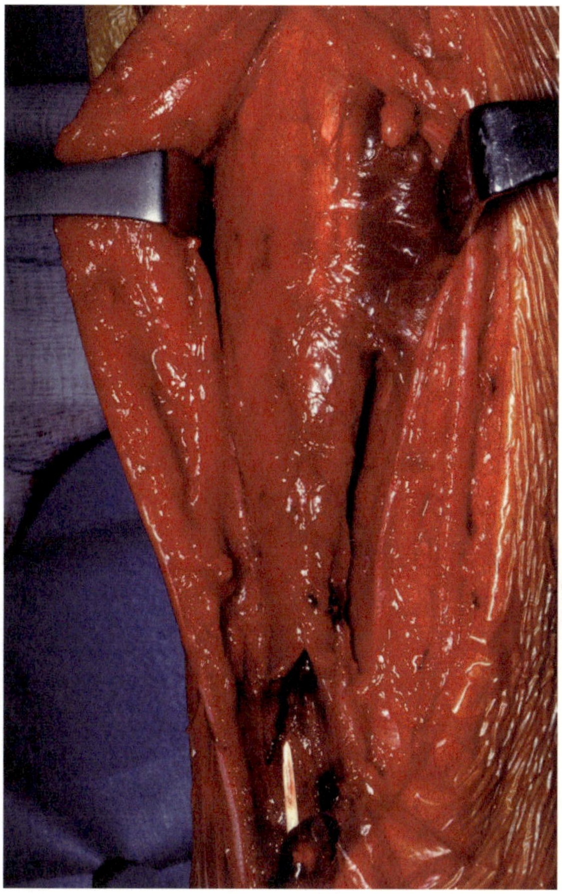

Fig. 3. Intraoperative photo showing large gap that exceeds the capability of end to end repair

1975). An alternative method of advancement is a tongue-in-groove configuration **[Figures 4-7]**. However, more recently the argument is made against greater than 5cm of advancement as this can lead to detachment from the underlying muscle and cause weakness and decreased peak torque in plantarflexion when compared to the uninjured side (Kissel et al., 1994; Us et al., 1997).

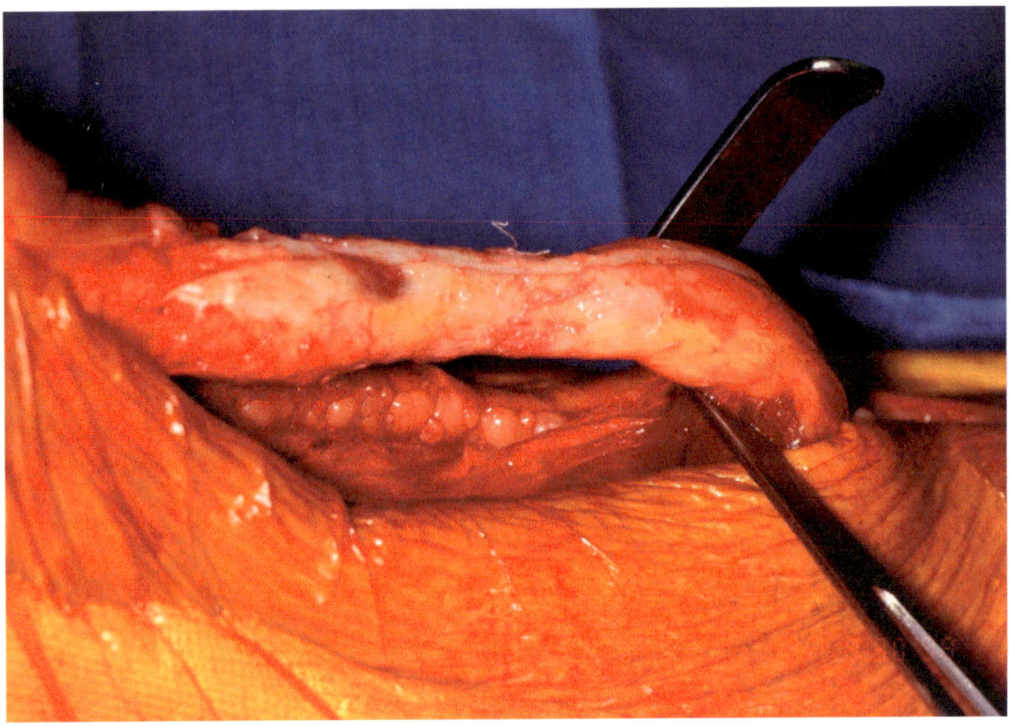

Fig. 4. Intraoperative photo showing interposed scar tissue in neglected rupture

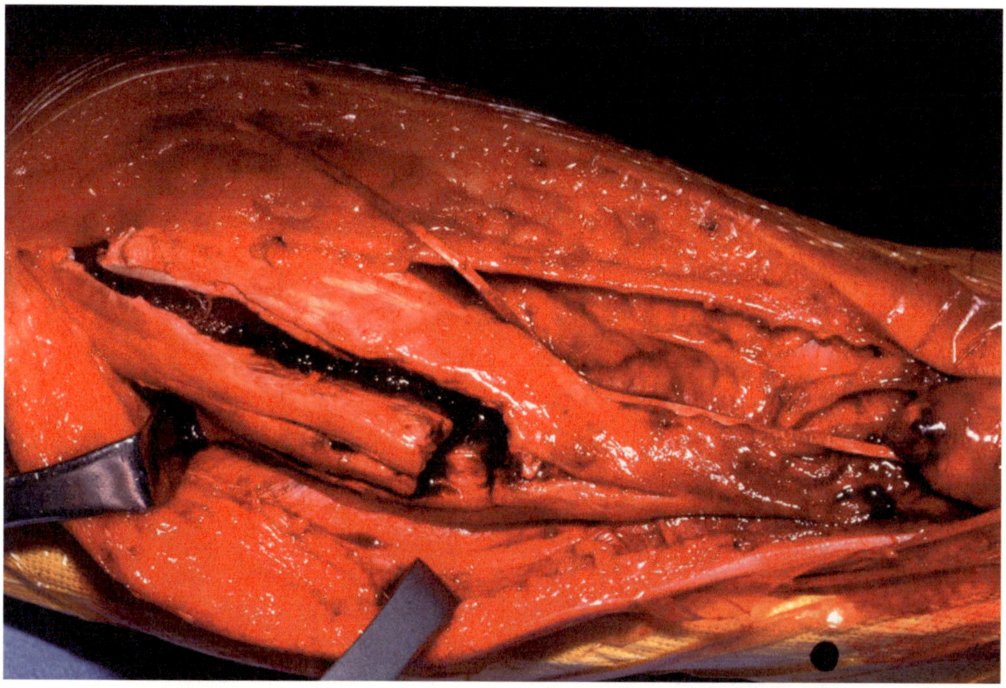

Fig. 5. More proximally a tongue-in-groove lengthening is performed to mobilize distally (right) in order to bridge the gap.

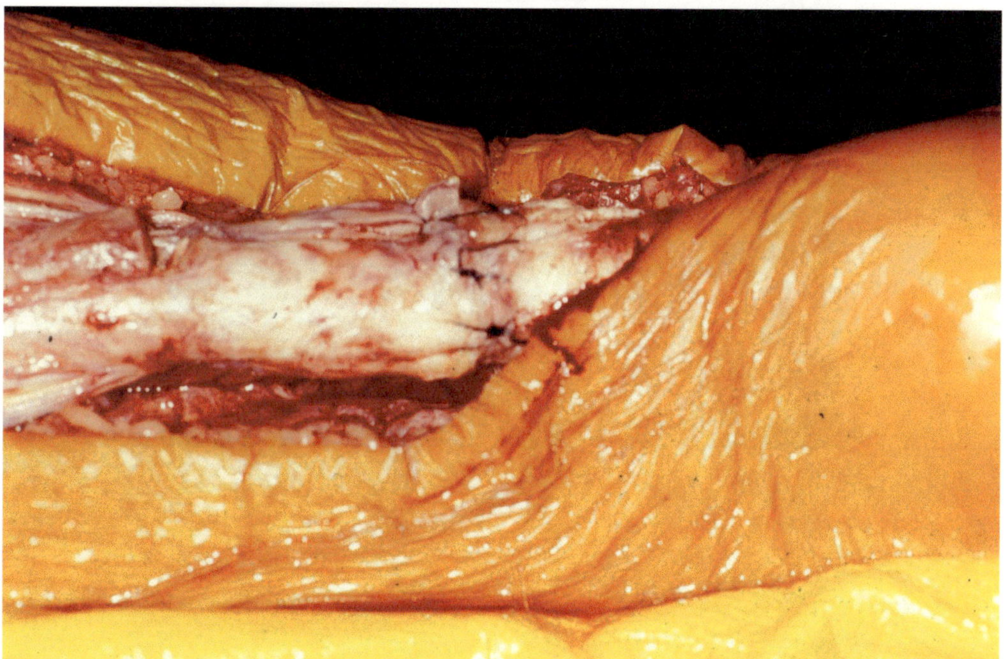

Fig. 6. The mobilized proximal portion of the gastrosoleal complex has been sutured to the distal stump of the Achilles.

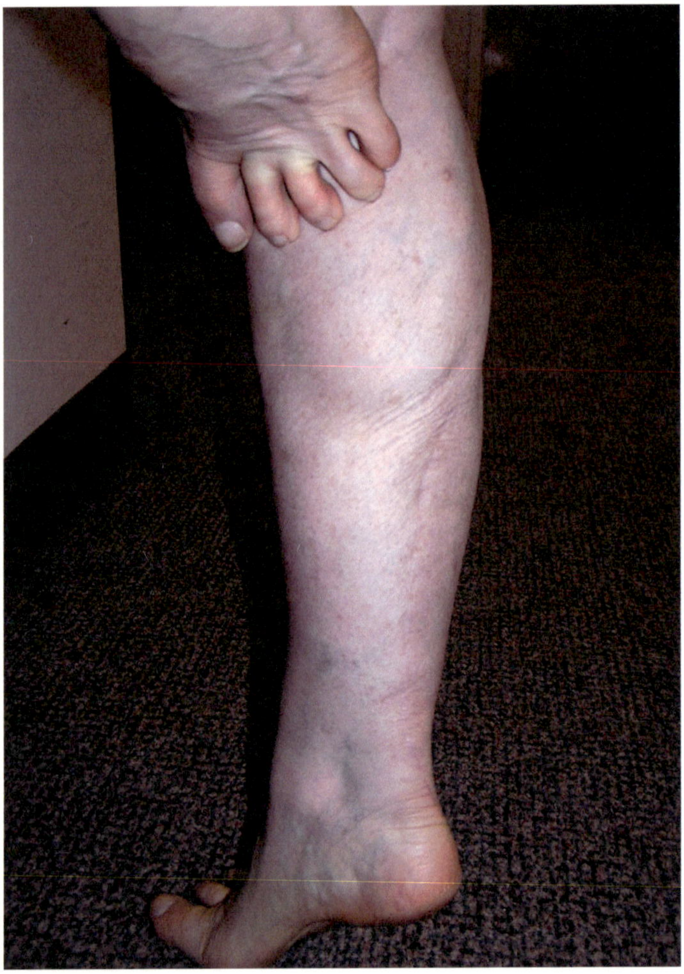

Fig. 7. At 6 months postoperative, the patient is able to do a single heel rise.

On many occasions direct primary repair is not feasible due to contracture of the ruptured tendon ends over time and a more extensive reconstructive effort is needed. In general, the longer the interval between injury and repair, the more likely primary repair will not be possible, even with mobilization of the proximal segment. When delayed primary repair is not possible, some surgeons advocate bridging of the gap with other augmentation methods at the site of the defect. The materials available for augmentation can be categorized into autologous, synthetic, or allograft augmentation techniques (Dalton, 1996). Several techniques with distant or local autologous tendon transfers have been described in order to reinforce or reconstruct neglected Achilles tendon rupture. Synthetic materials have also been used for augmentation. The advantage of using synthetic materials is that they avoid sacrificing other active tendons. In turn, the morbidity associated with larger incisions and dissections involved in autologous techniques can be bypassed. However, the use of synthetic materials in the area well-known for tenuous wound healing is a major disadvantage. More recently, Achilles tendon allografts have been used for reconstruction of neglected Achilles tendon rupture. The allograft technique can used to reconstruct large defects without sacrificing other autologous lower extremity tendons with relative technical ease.

Instead of advancement of the proximal gastrosoleal complex to negotiate the resultant gap, various gastrocnemius-soleus fascia turn-down techniques have been described. A longitudinal strip of the gastrocnemius fascia can be turned down with the distal end still attached. The 1.5 cm wide strip is then weaved in-out of the proximal and distal ruptured ends to bridge the gap (Bosworth, 1956). Other modifications of the turn down fascial flap have included the use of two flaps measuring 1 x 8 cm that are raised from the proximal gastrocnemius fascia. The distal portions of the flaps are left attached distally 3 cm proximal to the tendon end and turned 180 degrees on themselves. The flaps are sutured into the distal stump as well as to each other (Arner & Lindholm, 1959; Lindholm, 1959). Alternatively, a centrally based turn-down flap can be developed from the proximal segment which is then turned 180 degrees on itself and approximated to the distal stump (Coughlin et al, 2007). In this technique the proximal flap is passed deep to the proximal portion to decrease the bulk. Although these methods are useful in bridging the gap in continuity, strength deficits of up to 23% have been reported (Takao et al., 2003).

3.1 Free fascia-tendon graft

Several authors have reported on the use of free distant fascial or tendon grafts for the reconstruction of neglected ruptures (Maffulli et al., 2005) (Bugg & Boyd, 1968). Free tendinous autograft, utilizing a tongue-in-groove gastrocnemius recession has been described as well (Schuberth et al, 1984). Either the fascia lata or gracilis tendon can be utilized. The usual posterior approach is made and the scar tissue is excised. An ipsilateral incision is made in the thigh to harvest a section of fascia lata 7.5 by 15 cm in dimension. Three 1 cm wide sections are fashioned and laid across the defect between the tendon defects obliquely **[Figure 8]**. The remaining fascia lata is then wrapped around the repair with the serosal side facing outward (Bugg & Boyd, 1968). Maffulli et al used a free gracilis tendon graft in 21 patients with neglected ruptures. In a minimum follow up of 2 years, no re-ruptures were reported all patients were able to stand on tip-toes with no visible limp during gait. However, the calf circumference remained significantly reduced and the operative limb was significant weaker than the uninjured side at final review (Maffulli et al., 2005).

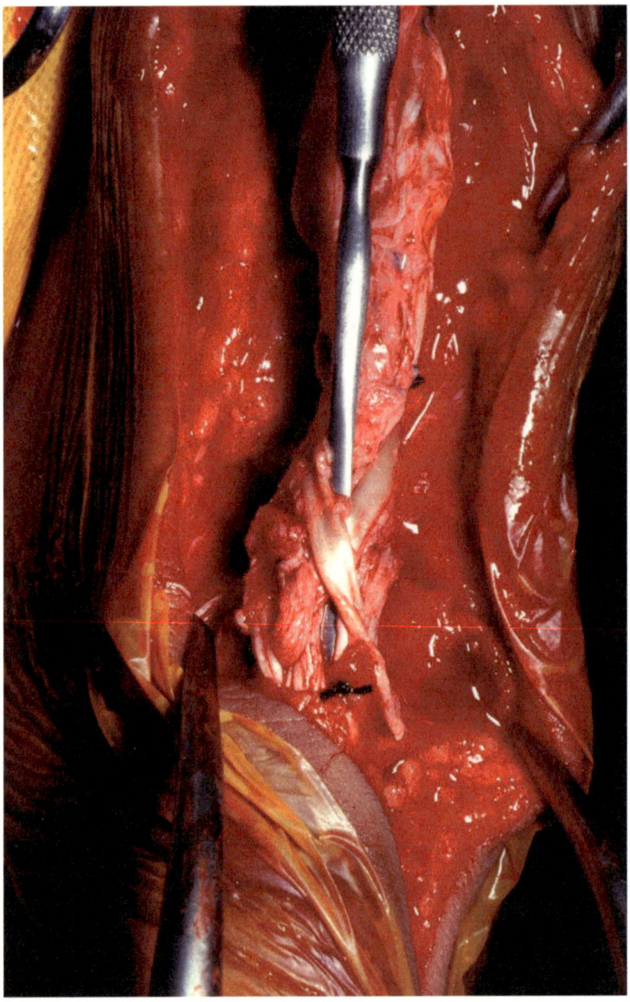

Fig. 8. Intraoperative photo showing strip of fascia lata rolled up and placed around repair site for augmentation.

3.2 Local tendon transfers

The increased technical difficulty of utilizing free tendon grafts as well as need for a separate incision has made local tendon transfers more popular. The use of a local tendon utilizes a viable structure with an intact vascular supply and can augment the plantar flexion strength. Although the biomechanical characteristics and caliber of the transferred tendon is dissimilar to that of the recipient, it can provide additional blood supply to the deficit and avoids the host rejection possible with the use of allografts. The current rule of thumb is to utilize tendon augmentation for defects greater than 2-3 cm (Den Hartog, 2008). The most commonly used are flexor hallucis longus (FHL) and flexor digitorum longus (FDL) tendons. Peroneus brevis (PB) tendon transfer has been utilized in both neglected and recurrent ruptures. (White & Kraynick, 1959; Schuberth, 1984). Plantaris and posterior tibial (PT) tendon transfers have been described as well (Schedl & Faso, 1979; Platt, 1931).

3.3 FHL tendon transfer

The use of FHL tendon has become popular in the repair of the neglected Achilles tendon rupture. In part it is due to the mechanical advantage compared to the other autologous transfers, as it has been shown to be stronger than the PB and almost twice as strong as the FDL tendon. Further, it is active during the same phase as the triceps surae complex and helps maintain normal ankle function (Pintore et al., 2001; Leppilahti & Orava, 1998; Den Hartog, 2008).The close proximity to the Achilles tendon affords a readily accessible harvest site. The abundant vascular supply to the muscle belly of the FHL extends to the distal avascular region of the Achilles tendon, improving the blood supply to the injured area (Wilcox et al., 2000; Wapner et al., 1993; Wapner et al, 1995; Carr & Norris, 1989; Martin et al., 2005; Monroe et al., 2000). The FHL tendon can be sewn to the Achilles in a side-to-side fashion, or transferred directly to the calcaneus. Good to excellent functional results have been reported even though there was a reduction in plantar flexion strength (Wapner et al., 1993). Similar good to excellent results were obtained in later studies utilizing the more proximal harvest (at the distal tip of the medial malleolus) in which the FHL tendon transfer was used after extensive debridement for chronic Achilles tendinosis (Den Hartog, 2003; Wilcox et al., 2000; Coull et al., 2003). The argument for using a separate medial incision to harvest the FHL tendon is to obtain the longest working length of the tendon possible. The average tendon length from the posterior incision was 5.16 cm compared to 8.09 cm that can be obtained from a separate medial incision (Tashjian et al., 2003). Although a much longer tendon can be harvested from a separate incision, the more proximal harvest was found be sufficient for transfer and solid fixation into the calcaneus. The loss of FHL function and alteration of the forefoot loading pattern have been shown to be minimal after FHL tendon transfers (Wapner et al., 1995; Coull et al., 2003). After FHL harvest, there is little pressure change to the plantar first or second metatarsophalangeal joint with no clinical functional deficit of the first ray (Coull et al., 2003).

The surgical exposure is approached through a posteromedial incision with the patient in prone position. Once the Achilles tendon is exposed and interposing scar tissue has been excised the deep fascia anterior to the Achilles tendon is incised to expose the FHL tendon and muscle belly. The tendon is then coursed through the fibro-osseous tunnel alongside the calcaneal tuberosity. The neurovascular bundle is in close proximity to the FHL tendon distally and should be protected. The great toe and the ankle are plantarflexed and the FHL tendon is cut from medial to lateral orientation as far distal as possible (Den Hartog, 2008; Hansen, 1991). The FHL tendon is then mobilized and assessed for sufficient length for transfer and the end of the tendon is secured with a Krackow stitch (Den Hartog, 2008; Grove & Hardy, 2008). Some advocate the resection of the superior aspect of the calcaneal tuberosity to create sufficient space for the FHL tendon (Den Hartog, 2008). The FHL tendon is placed under tension with the foot in 20 degrees of plantarflexion (Den Hartog, 2008). If sufficient length of the tendon is available an interference screw is used through drill in the calcaneus. Suture anchors can also be used if the length of the harvested tendon is too short for the interference technique (Den Hartog, 2008).

3.4 PB tendon transfer

The routine use of peroneus brevis is not widely practiced because of the loss of eversion and presumed frontal plane stability. Although subjectively, there seems to be a loss of eversion power, the loss of ankle stability does not seem to develop as a consequence

(Gallant et al. 1995) (Miskulin, 2005). In addition, the availability of other autologous options has made the use of this tendon almost obsolete. Historically PB tendon transfer has been described in repairing acute Achilles tendon ruptures (Teuffer, 1974). Later, there were reports of good to excellent results using this technique in cases with large defects in tendon continuity or poor quality tissue (Hepp & Blauth, 1978) (Schuberth, 1984). No obvious functional deficits secondary to the loss of the function of the PB tendon were noted.

The published reports regarding the use of PB tendon in the treatment of neglected rupture of the Achilles tendon have generally noted good functional results. (White & Kraynick, 1959) (Miskulin, 2005). Miskulin et al performed PB tendon transfer in conjunction with plantaris tendon augmentation in 5 patients with neglected rupture with an average of 19.8 weeks (range 5-40 weeks) of delay in injury to presentation. They found that all 5 patients were able to return to pre-injury activity level. There were no reported wound complications, postoperative pain, or function limitations. Using an isokinetic dynamometer, they found that all 5 patients had increase in peak plantarflexion torque approximately 1 year after surgery and all were able to perform single toe rise on the involved side after the reconstruction.

Surgical exposure is obtained through a posterolateral incision. The sural nerve is identified and protected throughout the procedure. The deep fascia is then incised and the PB muscle belly with the tendon is visualized. The interposing scar tissue is resected from the ruptured ends of the Achilles tendon. In order the harvest the PB tendon distally a separate incision is made (1 cm to 1.5 cm) directly over the base of the fifth metatarsal. The tendon is transected at this point and pulled through the original posterolateral incision. The foot is then plantarflexed 20 degrees and end-to-end anastomosis is attempted when feasible. Some use the plantaris tendon to augment the primary anastomosis. If the distal stump of the Achilles tendon appears to be in good condition the PB tendon is pulled through the distal stump (lateral to medial) and sutured to the proximal and the distal tendon stumps. It can also be secured to the calcaneus with an interference screw or suture anchors (Miskulin, 2005).

3.5 FDL tendon transfer

The use of FDL tendon has been advocated as it mimics the course of the Achilles tendon without comprising the lesser digit function postoperatively. There use of this tendon also avoids the loss of eversion and ankle balance seen with transfer of the PB. Mann et al first described the technique in 7 patients with duration of symptoms ranging from 3 to 36 months with an average follow up of 39 months. They achieved excellent result in 4 patients, good in 2, and fair in 1. The 6 patients who achieved good to excellent result were all able to return to pre-injury activities without pain. Two patients with good result had wound complications requiring a secondary procedure. No re-ruptures were reported in their series and active plantarflexion of the digits were preserved and no hammer-toe deformities were seen postoperatively (Mann et al., 1991). The exposure involves a hockey stick shaped incision beginning medial to the Achilles tendon and continues distally to the insertion. The incision is curved laterally to expose the entire Achilles tendon unit. A second linear incision is made just distal and inferior to the navicular tuberosity but superior to the abductor hallucis muscle. The abductor hallucis muscle is retracted plantarly and the FHL, FDL, and FHB (flexor hallucis brevis) tendons are identified. The master knot of Henry can be released in order to improve the visualization of the tendons. The FDL tendon is identified proximal to the division to digital branches and resected. The proximal aspect of the distal FDL tendon segment is then sutured to the FHL tendon while the digits are held with the interphalangeal joints in neutral position. If the patient had pre-existing hammer-toe deformities, the distal portion can be left free. The FDL tendon is then freed and pulled through the original posterior incision. The tendon sheath is incised and the transferred tendon is placed next to the Achilles tendon. A drill hole is made in the posterior aspect of the calcaneus and the tendon is passed through from medial to lateral and sutured onto itself while the foot is held in 10 to 15 degrees of plantarflexion. If fortification of the tendon interface is deemed necessary, a central slip from the proximal Achilles stump is mobilized and flipped distally and cross-sutured to the FDL tendon and the distal stump (Mann et al., 1991).

3.6 Fascia advancement in conjunction with local tendon transfer

Recently FHL tendon transfer in conjunction with fascia advancement has been advocated for neglected ruptures with defects greater than 5 cm (Elias, 2007; Den Hartog, 2008). The argument for the combined procedures is that fascia advancement, whether in forms of turn-down flap, V-Y plasty, etc., provides continuity of the Achilles tendon while the transferred tendon can provide plantarflexory power. Elias et al. reported on 15 patients with a neglected rupture that underwent a FHL tendon transfer in conjunction with a V-Y plasty with an average follow-up of 106 weeks. Subjectively all patients were satisfied with the outcome. No re-ruptures were reported in their series. The authors concluded that their result is at least comparable to previous studies in which fascial advancement or a FHL tendon transfer was performed alone.

3.7 Allograft

3.7.1 Achilles tendon allograft

Tendon allograft has become popular especially for the reconstructive knee and shoulder surgery. Achilles tendon allografts have shown to be effective in anterior cruciate ligament (ACL) reconstruction with similar functional outcomes compared to autografts. (Poehling et al., 2005; Indelli et al., 2004). The use of Achilles tendon allograft for reconstruction of the neglected Achilles ruptures have been reported but mostly limited to case reports (Nellas et al., 1996; Yuen & Nicholas, 2000; Lepow & Green, 2006). All authors reported favorable outcome after the operation. The use of allograft has been recommended when significant segmental defect is encountered, such as, greater than 10 cm when fascia advancement or tendon transfer is not able to provide sufficient bridging between the tendon ends (Den Hartog, 2008; Lepow, 2006). The use of an allograft allows bridging of a large tendon defect with an adequate graft, avoidance of donor site morbidity, and relative ease of surgical technique. However, any allograft carries the small risk of transmission of disease and graft rejection by the host. The risk of viral disease transmission has been shown to be low, however, with the most recent report by the American Association of Tissue Banks showing no incidence of viral disease transmission in more than 2 million musculoskeletal allografts distributed within 5 years at the time of the report (Mahirogullari et al., 2007). In addition, functional outcomes over a long follow-up period have not been established.

In an animal study the mechanical strength of an allograft tendon is similar to that of an autograft (Mahirogullari et al, 2007). However, the maturation process (remodeling) is longer for the allograft and it is this phase that the tendon is most vulnerable to injury (Lepow & Green, 2006). This process has been shown to vary from 26 weeks to 18 months in animal studies (Shino et al., 1998; Arnoczky et al., 1986., Jackson et al., 1987). The allograft serves as a scaffold for remodeling and once the maturation process is complete, histological studies have shown similar cellular composition to a native tendon (Drez et al., 1991). However, the correlation of this process with the return to normal function has yet to be established.

The surgical approach is made through the standard posteromedial incision with the patient in the prone position. A surgical plane is created between the subcutaneous tissue and the paratenon which is then incised. All fibrotic tissue interposed between the ruptured ends is resected until normal appearing tendon is visualized on both ends of the native tendon **[Figure 9]**. The Achilles allograft is thawed and rehydrated in sterile normal saline solution for 30 minutes prior to insertion. The graft is cut to the appropriate size to fill defect with the

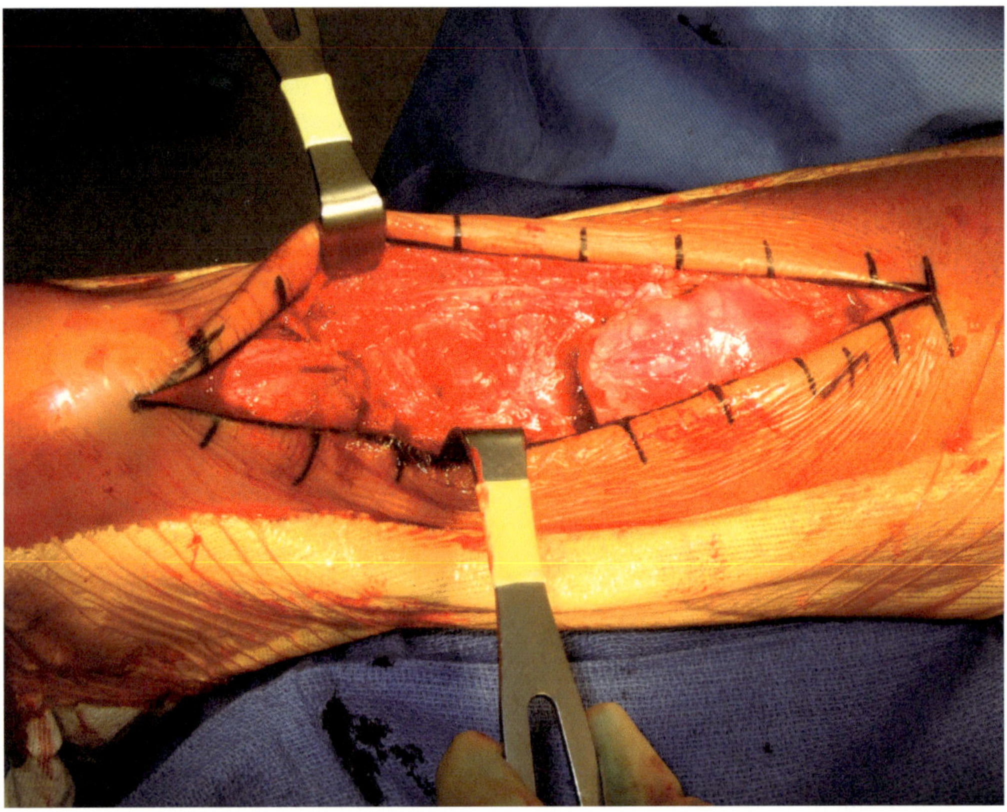

Fig. 9. All fibrotic tissue has been debrided in this neglected rupture, creating a large defect.

foot in approximately 20 degrees of plantarflexion **[Figures 10-11]**. The suturing technique can vary depending on the surgeon's preference. Common tendon suture such as a running Krackow, Kessler or modified Bunnel stitch are used at either end to secure the allograft. Proximally the allograft gastrocnemius aponeurosis is placed over the native aponeurosis prior to suturing. Distally, the allograft comes with attached portion of a calcaneus and in cases where the distal tendon end is insufficient for repair, the calcaneal portion can be fixed to the recipient calcaneus with either some drill holes from dorsal to plantar at the insertion site **[Figure 12]** or with an inset technique using the allograft bone portion and internal fixation at the insertion site **[Figures 13-14]**.

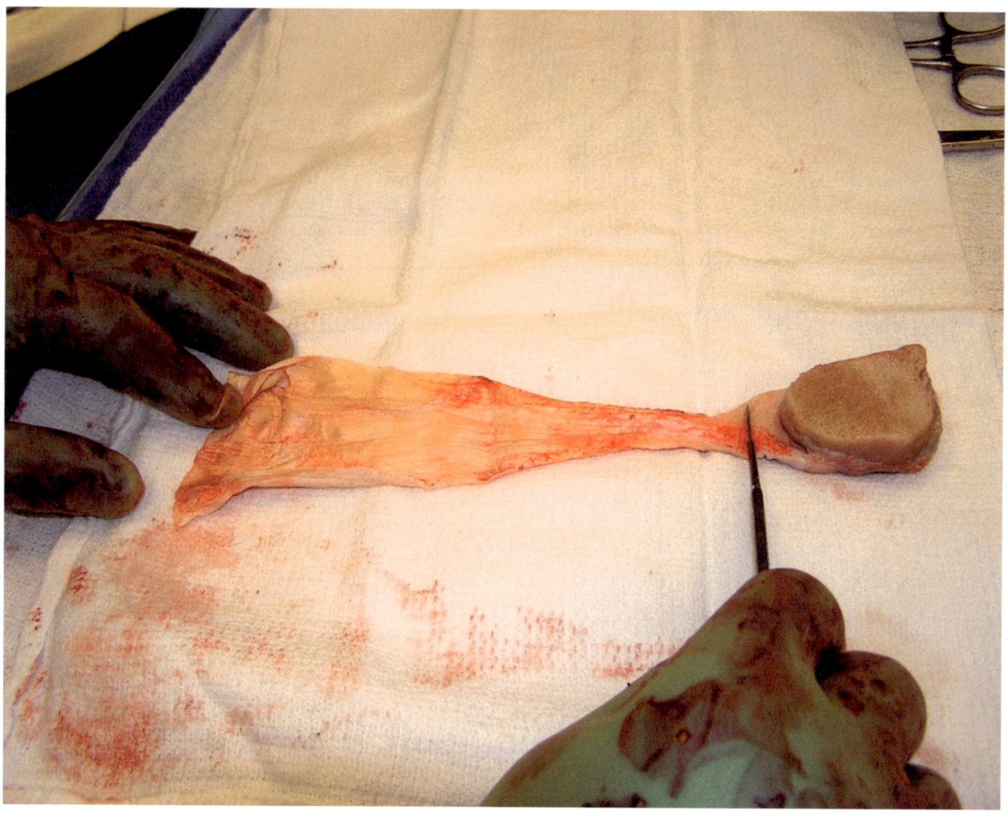

Fig. 10. The Achilles tendon allograft with attached bone is being prepared for insertion

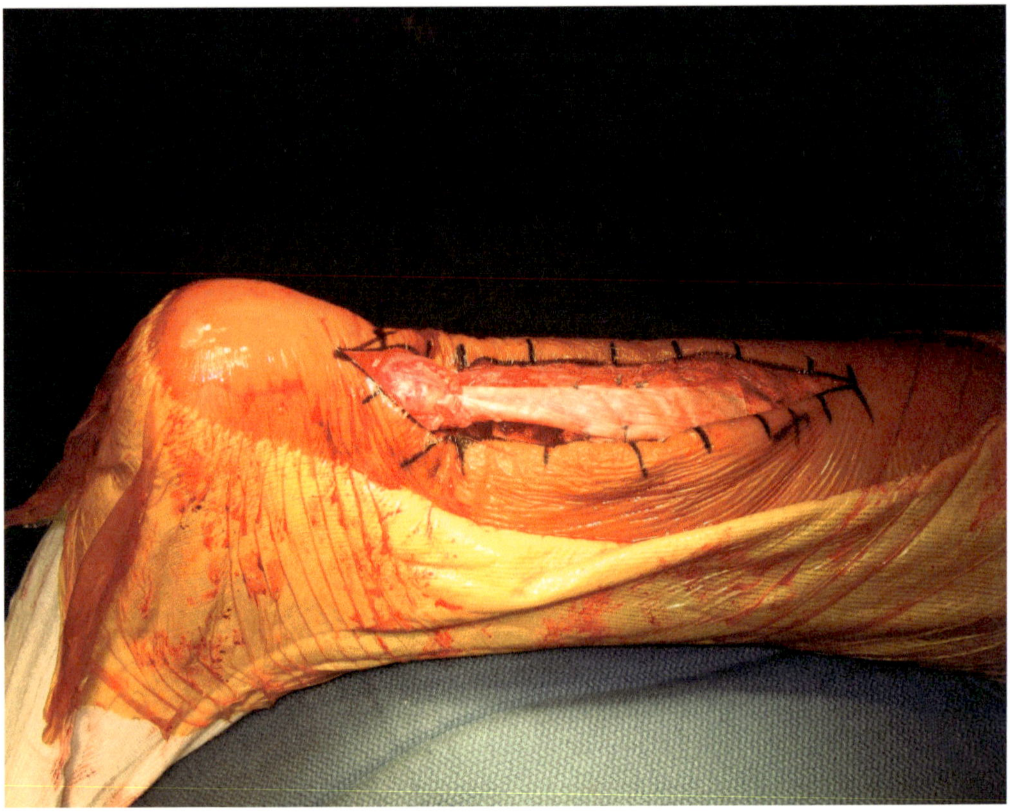

Fig. 11. The allograft Achilles tendon is sewn into place with the appropriate amount of tension.

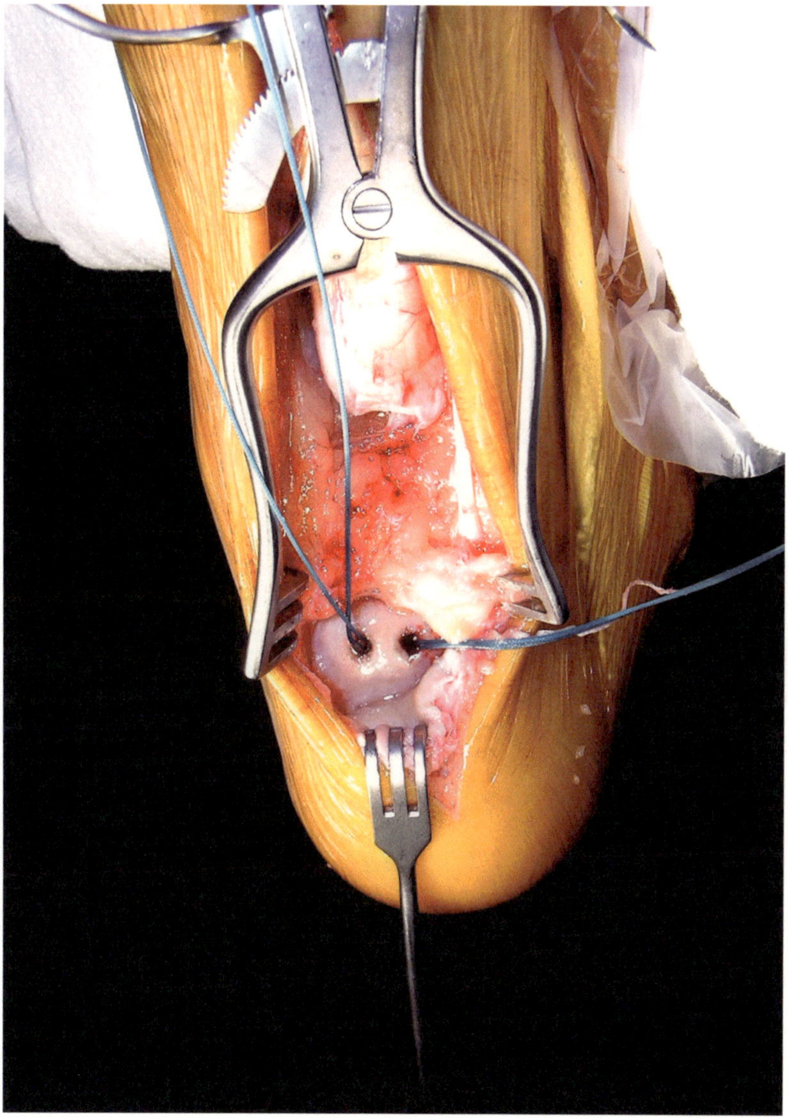

Fig. 12. The dorsal aspect of the calcaneus has been prepared with drill holes to accept sutures for anchoring of the allograft to the bone.

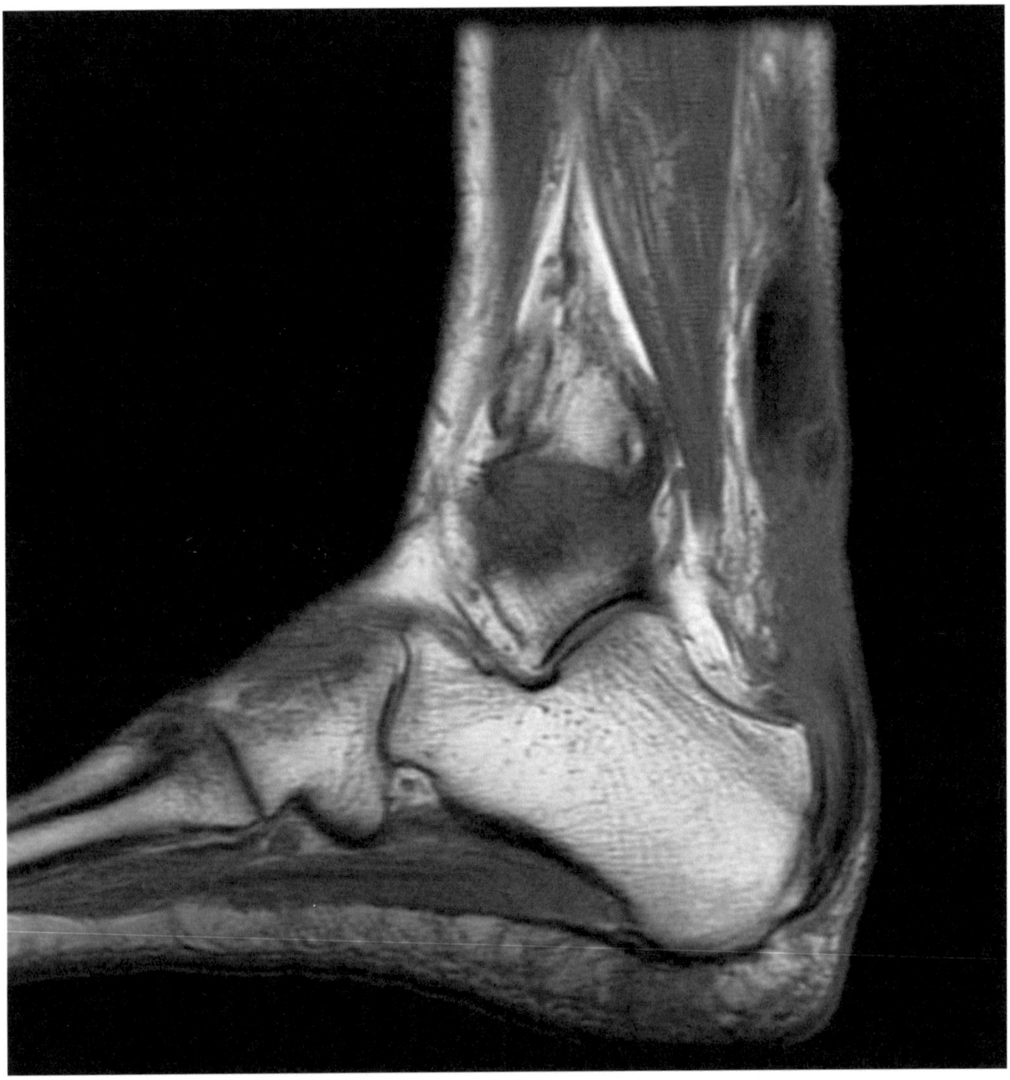

Fig. 13. MRI with insufficient Achilles tendon at the calcaneus.

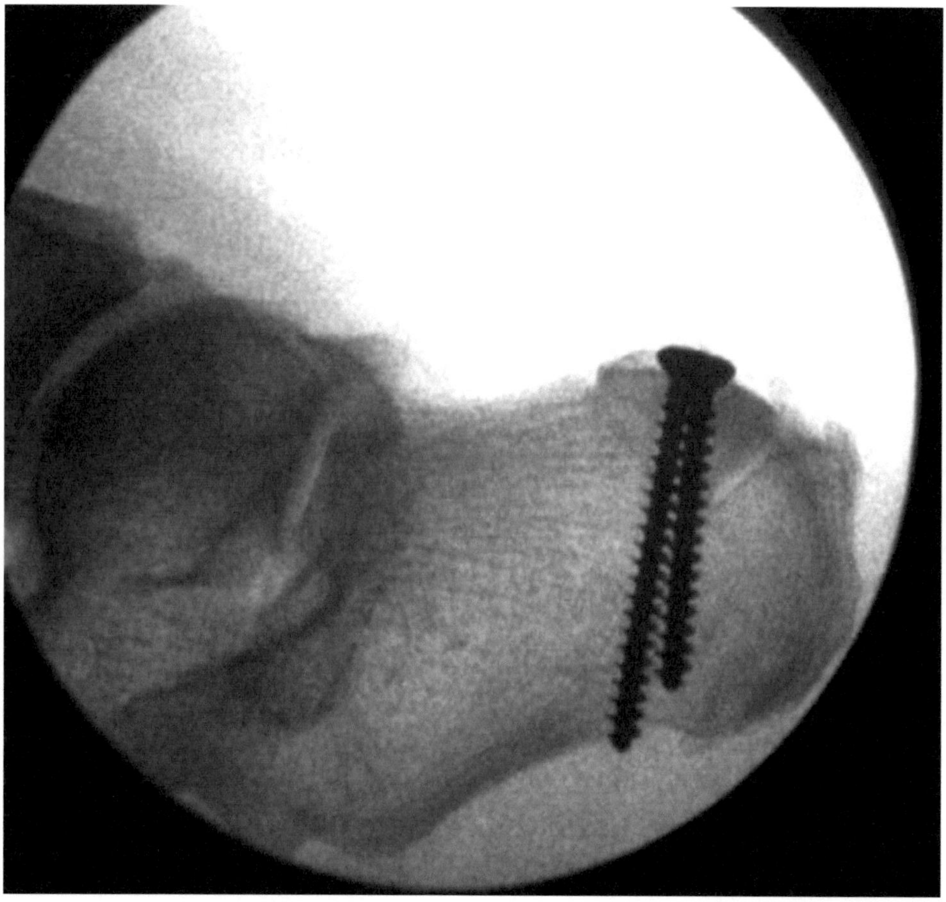

Fig. 14. Technique showing utilization of bone block with the Achilles tendon allograft. (Courtesy of David Deng, DPM)

3.7.2 Synthetic grafts

Several synthetic materials have been used with success in some early studies. These materials include vascular grafts, carbon fiber composites, polyglycol threads, and polyester mesh (Lieberman et al, 1988; Parsons et al, 1989; Shedl & Fasol, 1979; Ozaki et al., 1989). The use of synthetic materials avoids the sacrifice of functional tendon structures and extensive incision and dissection. Foreign body reaction has been observed with the use of carbon or polyester fiber (Amis et al., 1984). However, the introduction of a foreign material into an area notorious for tenuous healing makes the use of a synthetic graft unfavorable. Unlike synthetic grafts, an acellular dermal matrix graft has been shown in animal studies to be able to b incorporate into the native tissue and resemble autologous tendon histologically (Mandelbaum et al., 1995). Lee in 2007 reported on 9 patients who underwent primary repair of a neglected Achilles rupture with augmentation by an acellular dermal matrix graft. The follow-up ranged from 20 to 30 months with no incidence of re-rupture. All patients were able to perform single heel raise on the reconstructed side (Lee, 2007).

4. Complications of surgical treatment

Although most operations result in reasonably successful and functional outcomes, significant complications can occur. One of the variables during surgical reconstruction is determining the optimal tension of the repaired tendon. If the tendon complex is too tight, then the patient will have some difficulty in attaining a plantigrade foot. Extensive physical therapy in the postoperative period may diminish some of the equinus position but generally the resultant deformity is not easily treated because the resultant scar tissue that forms in the gap has a more limited capacity to stretch than native tissue. The collagen structure is more loosely organized with irregular cross-linking, resulting in a less resilient tendon.

On the other hand, the reconstructed tendon may have healed in a lengthened position which causes some functional weakness. The ultimate determinant of a good result is the capability to do a single limb heel-rise. In most cases, this is attainable around 6 months postoperatively but will not be possible if the tendon reconstruction has too much laxity and not enough tension. The patient may complain of weakness particularly on hills, but on physical exam there is a distinct asymmetry with the affected leg assuming a more dorsiflexed posture in the prone position **[Figure 15]**.

One way to avoid this complication during the repair is to match the position of the unaffected leg intraoperatively. Often this requires that the unaffected leg be draped free as well for comparison. Modulation of the position is actually easier in the neglected rupture because the tendon is not frayed and more accurate purchase of the tissues by the suture allows for better control of the length. If however, the patient has unacceptable weakness, a shortening of the reconstructed tendon can be performed **[Figures 16-17]**.

Although the incidence of rerupture is far less after repair of a neglected rupture compared to repair of the acute rupture, the incidence is not zero. Given the high tensile strength sutures available today, the failure point is almost always at the suture tissue junction rather than a failure of the suture material. From a speculative standpoint, the quality of tissue after a negelected rupture is not as robust and may handle the tension from sutures poorly. Other possibilities of failure include the unraveling of the suture material due to the slippery nature of the knot. **[Figure 18]**.

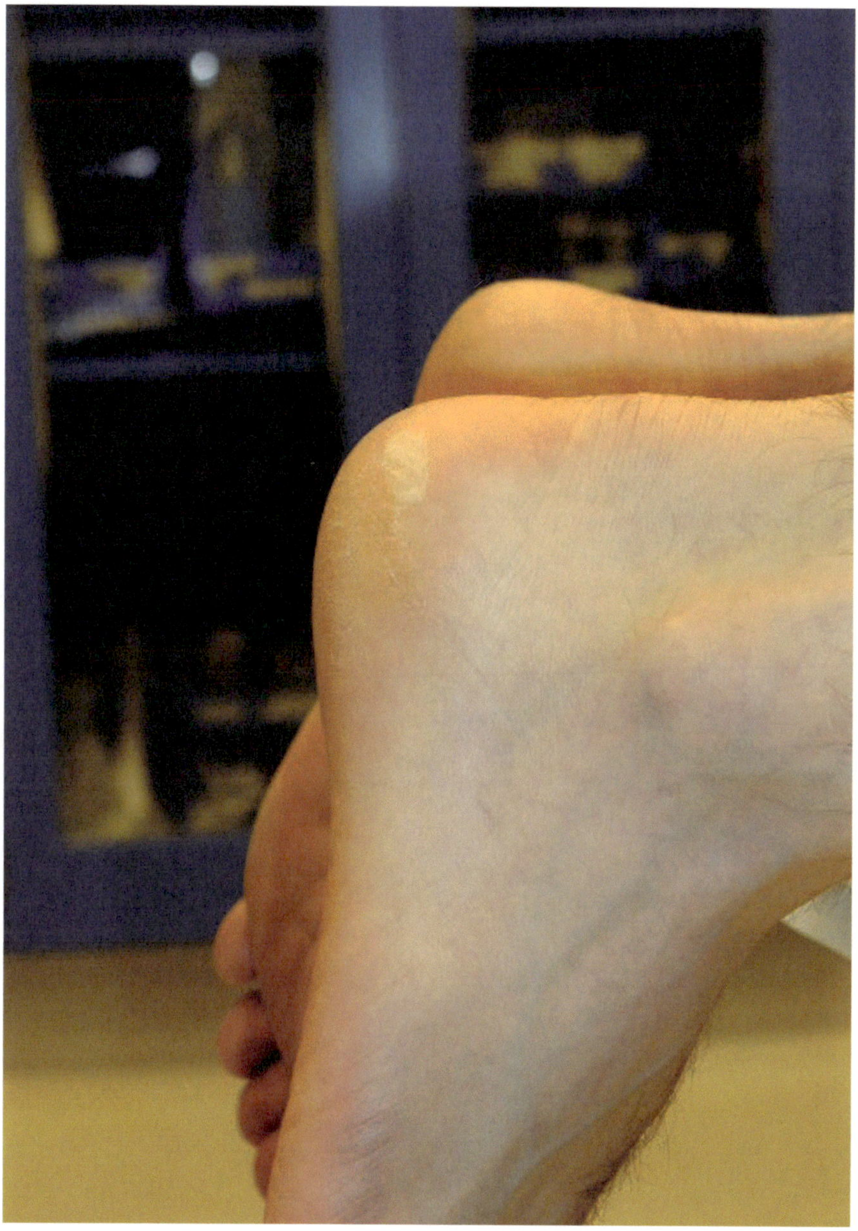

Fig. 15. Postoperative result after repair of delayed rupture. Note the accentuated on the right side.

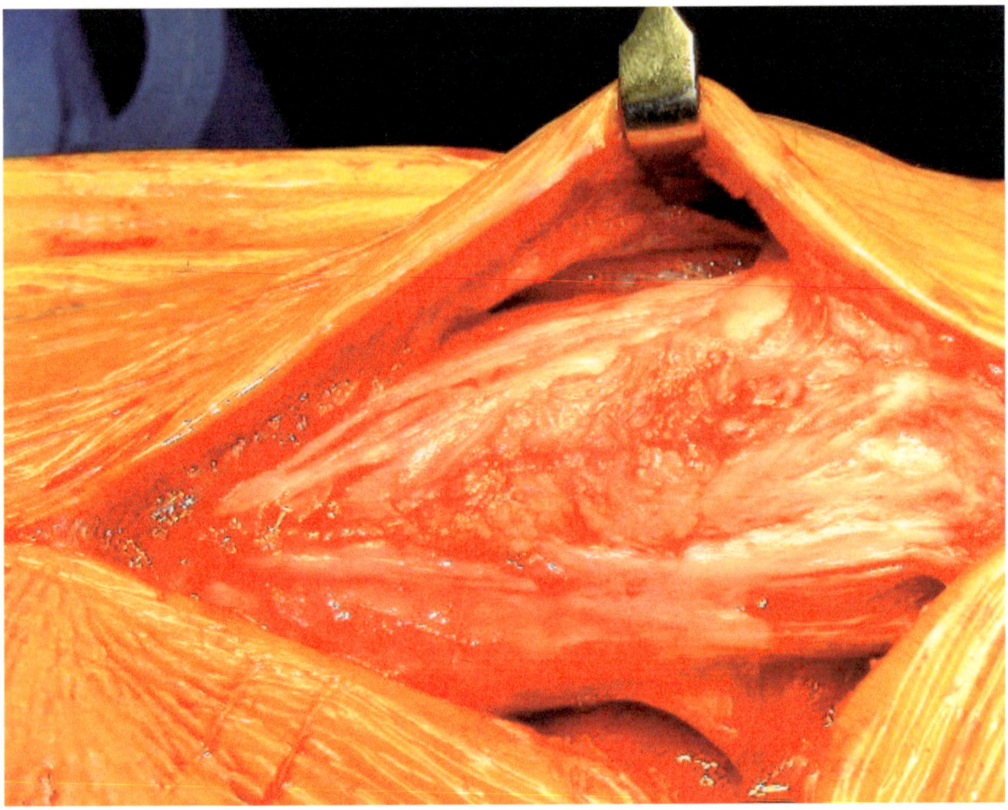

Fig. 16. Intraoperative photo of overlengthened Achilles repair of a neglected rupture.

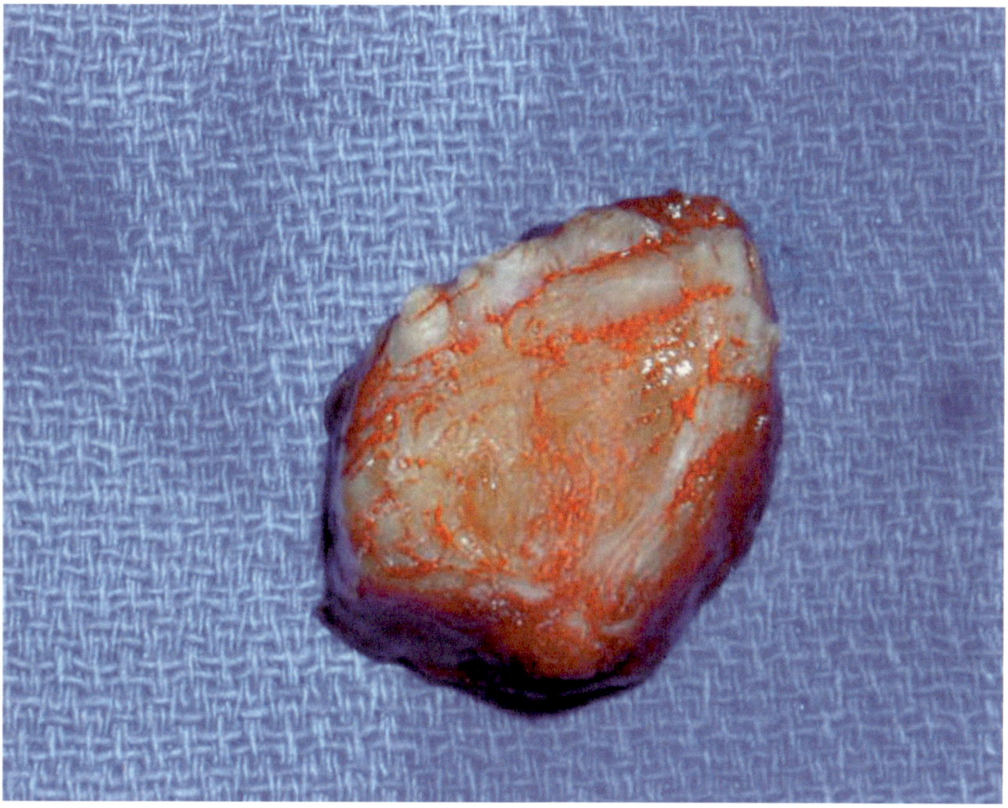

Fig. 17. Cylinder of resected tissue to correct for overlenghtening.

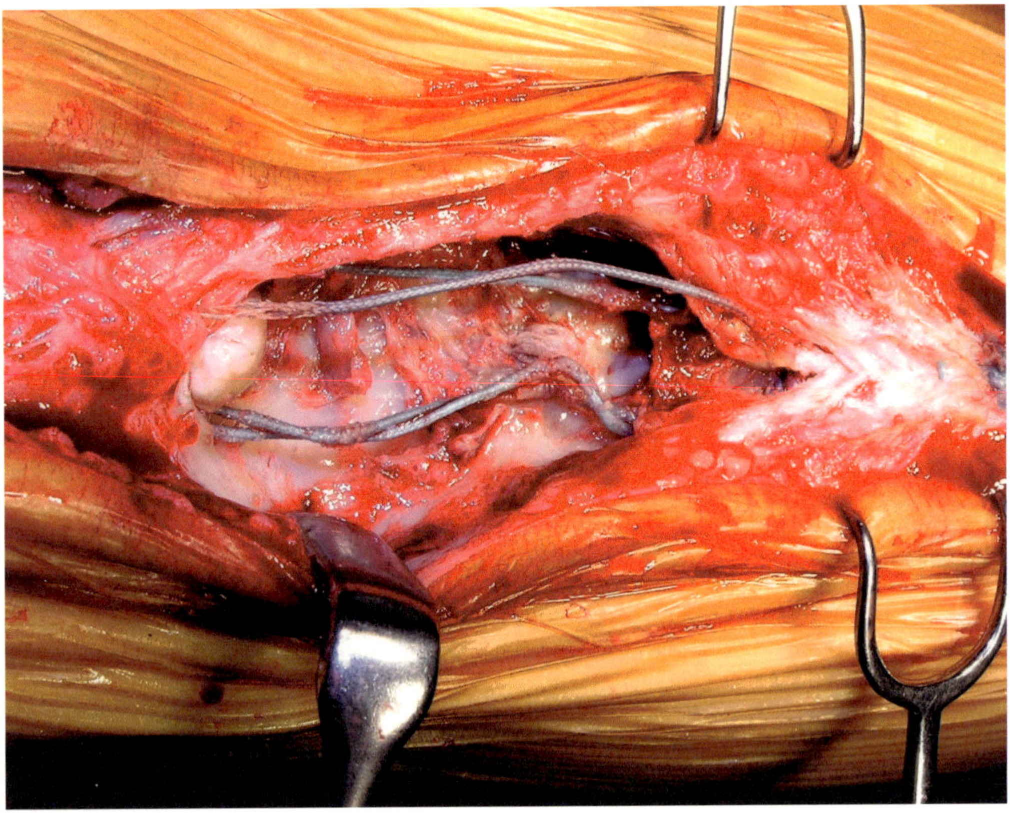

Fig. 18. Rerutpure after failure of the suture knot.

Wound problems are not uncommon after the repair of a neglected rupture. The local blood supply to the posterior aspect of the leg is often precarious and may be further disrupted by surgical intervention, introduction of foreign material such as allograft and the denser scar tissue that diminishes the healing capability of the skin **[Figures 19-20]**. Generally surgical exposures are more extensive compared to repair of the acute rupture, which also increases the chance of wound problems.

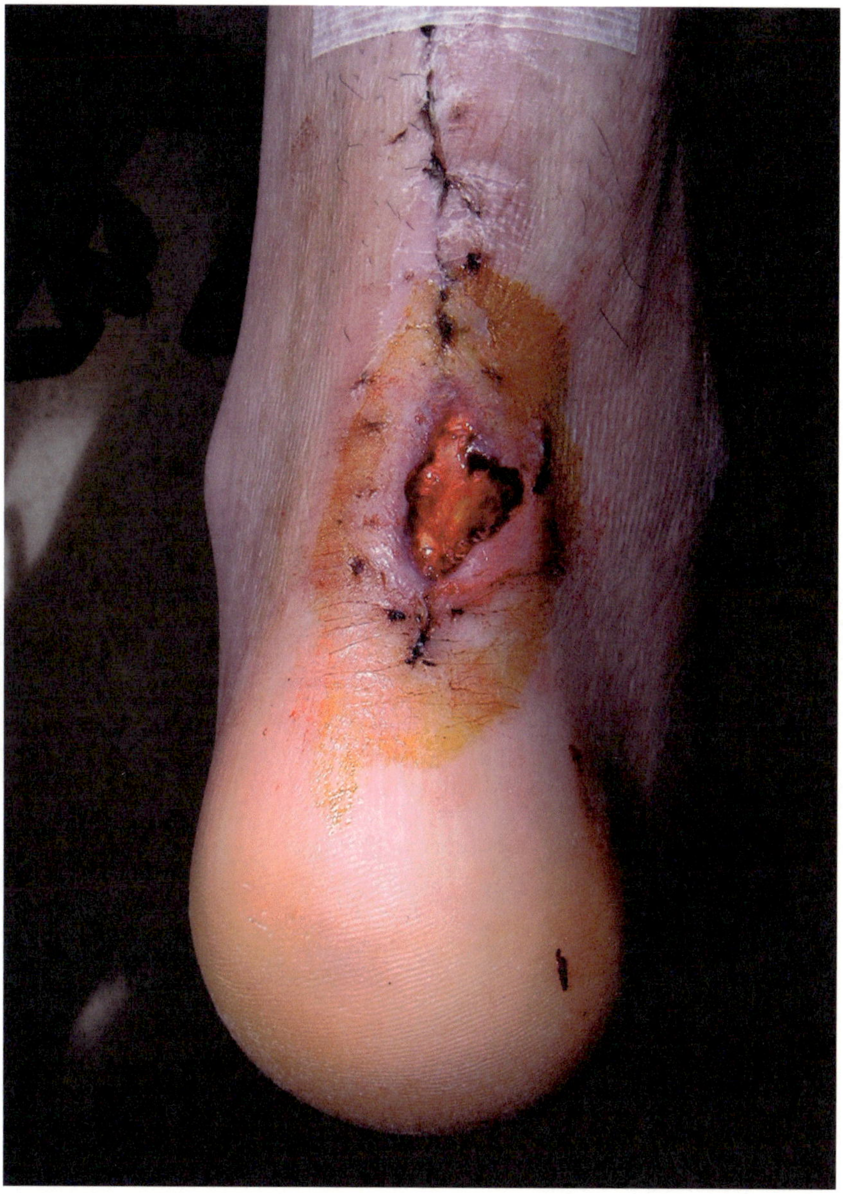

Fig. 19. Full thickness skin loss 4 weeks after routine repair of neglected rupture using a local gastrocnemius recession for tendon apposition.

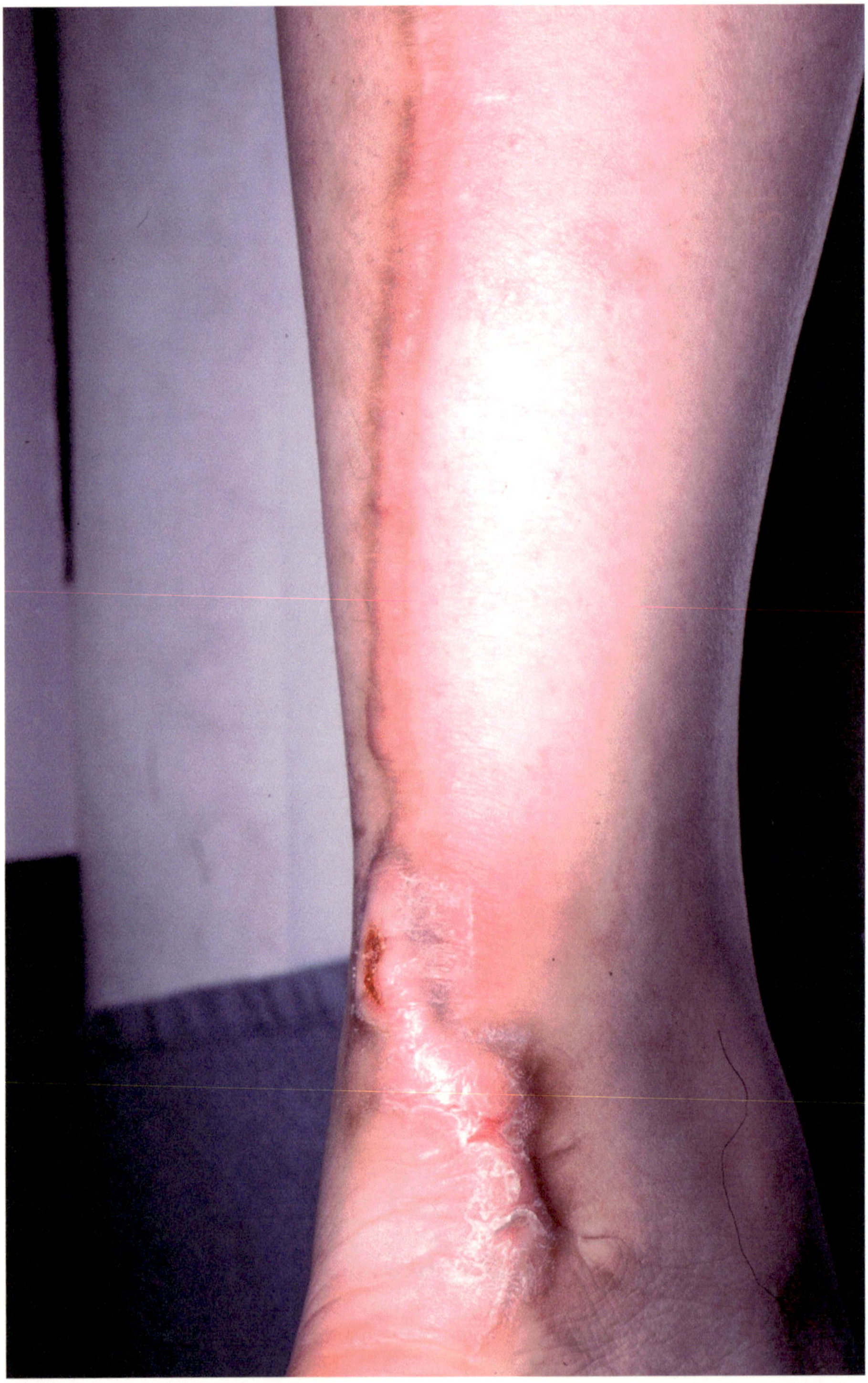

Fig. 20. Markedly hypertrophic scar after delayed operative repair of ruptured Achilles tendon

5. Conclusion

Many surgical treatments are available for reconstruction of a neglected Achilles tendon rupture. There is no concrete data to support one technique over another; hence, there is no "gold standard". Most agree, however, in order to achieve the optimal functional outcome surgical reconstruction is required. Regardless of the chosen technique, the ultimate goal of surgical treatment is to restore the length tension relationship such that sufficient plantar flexion power is attained. The ability of the patient to achieve a single limb heel rise on the affected side, most often indicates a successful outcome, although some patients are satisfied without attaining this goal.

Patients who have sufficient risk factors and/or low functional capacity may be better treated with bracing as local and more global surgical complications from reconstruction can be devastating (Boyden et al., 1995). The physician needs to decide on the proper treatment course appropriate for the individual patient. The length of the delay, risk factors, desired outcome, and functional requirement of each patient should be taken into account in implementing the appropriate treatment.

6. References

Abraham, E. & Pankovich, A. (1975). Neglected rupture of the Achilles tendon. Treatment by V-Y tendinous flap. *J Bone Joint Surg*, 57A, pp. 253- 255

Amis, A.; Campbell, J.; Kempson, S. & Miller, J. (1984). Comparison of the structure of neotendons induced by implantation of carbon or polyester fiber. *J Bone Joint Surg*, 66B, pp. 131-139

Anzel, S.; Covey, K.; Weiner. A. & Lipscomb, P (1959). Disruption of muscles and tendons; an analysis of 1,1014 cases. *Surgery*, 45, 3, pp. 406-414

Arner, O. & Lindholm, A. (1959). Subcutaneous rupture of the Achilles tendon; a study of 92 cases. *Acta Chir Scand*, 116, supp 239, pp. 1-51

Arnoczky, S.; Warren, R. & Ashlock, M. (1986). Replacement of the anterior cruciate ligament using a patellar tendon allograft: an experimental study. *J Bone Joint Surg Am*, 68, pp. 376 -385

Barnes, M. & Hardy, A. (1986). Delayed reconstruction of the calcaneal tendon. *J Bone Joint Surg Br*, 68, 1, pp. 121-124

Bosworth, D. (1956). Repair of defects in the tendo achillis. *J Bone Joint Surg Am*, 38-A, 1, pp. 111-114

Boyden, E.; Kitaoka, H.; Cahalan, T. & An, K. (1995). Late versus early repair of Achilles tendon rupture. Clinical and biomechanical evaluation. *Clin Orthop Relat Res*, 317, pp. 150-158

Bugg, E. Jr. & Boyd, B. (1968). Repair of neglected rupture or laceration of the Achilles tendon.*Clin Orthop Relat Res*, 56, pp. 73-75

Carden, D.; Noble, J.; Chalmers, J.; Lunn, P. & Ellis, J. (1987). Rupture of the calcaneal tendon. The early and late management. *J Bone Joint Surg Br*, 69, 3, pp. 416-20

Carr, A. & Norris, S. (1989). The bood supply of the calcaneal tendon. *J Bone Joint Surg*, 71B, pp. 100-101

Cetti, R.; Christensen, S. & Ejsted, R. et al (1993). Operative versus non-operative treatment of Achilles tendon rupture. A prospective randomized study and review of the literature. *Am J Sports Med*, 21, 6, pp. 791-799

Christensen, I. (1953). Rupture of the Achilles tendon: analysis of 57 cases. *Acta Chir. Scand*, 106, pp. 50-60

Coughlin, M.; Mann, R. & Saltzman, C. (2007): Disorders of tendons, In: *Surgery of the foot and ankle, Eighth Edition*, pp. 1249-1261, Mosby, Inc., Philadelphia

Coull, R.; Flavin, R. & Stephens, M. (2003). Flexor hallucis longus tendon transfer: Evaluation of postoperative morbidity. *Foot Ankle Int*, 24, 12, pp. 931-934

Dalton, G. (1996). Achilles tendon rupture. *Foot Ankle Clin*, 1, pp. 225-236

Den Hartog, B. (2003). Flexor Hallucis Longus Tendon Transfer for Chronic Achilles Tendinosis. *Foot Ankle Int*, 24, 3, pp. 233 - 237

Drez, D. Jr.; DeLee, J.; Holden, J.; Arnoczky, S.; Noyes, F. & Roberts, T. (1991). Anterior cruciate ligament reconstruction using bone-patellar tendonbone allografts: a biological and biomechanical evaluation in goats. *Am J Sports Med*, 19, pp. 256 -263

Elias, I.; Besser, M.; Nazarian, L. & Rankin, S. (2007). Reconstruction for missed or neglected Achilles tendon rupture with V-Y lengthening and flexor hallucis longus tendon transfer through one incision. *Foot Ankle Int*, ,28, 12, pp. 1238-1248

Gallant, G.; Massie, C. & Turco, V. (1995). Assessment of eversion and plantarflexion strength after repair of the Achilles tendon rupture using peroneus brevis tendon transfer. *Am J Orthop*, 24, pp. 257–261

Grove, J. & Hardy, M. (2008). Autograft, allograft, and xenograft options in the treatment of neglected Achilles tendon ruptures: a historical review with illustration of surgical repair, In: The Foot and Ankle Online Journal, Available from: http://faoj.files.wordpress.com/2008/04/autograft-allograft-and-xenograft-options-in-treatment-of-neglected-achilles-tendon-ruptures.pdf

Habusta, S. (1995). Bilateral simultaneous rupture of the Achilles tendon. A rare traumatic injury. *Clin Orthop Relat Res*, 320, pp. 231-234

Hansen, S. (1991): Trauma to the Heel Cord, In: *Disorders of the Foot and Ankle, Second Edition*, Jahss, M., pp. 2357, W.B. Saunders, Philadelphia

Hepp, W. & Blauth, W. (1978). Zur Behandlung von Achilessehnendefekten mitder "peronaeus-brevis-plastik". *Arch Orth Traum Surg*, 9, pp. 195–200

Indelli, P.; Dillingham, M.; Fanton, G. & Schurman, D. (2004). Anterior cruciate ligament reconstruction using cryopreserved allografts. *Clin Orthop*, 420, pp. 268 –275

Jackson, D.; Grood, E.; Arnoczky, S.; Butler, D. & Simon, T. (1987). Freeze-dried anterior cruciate ligament with freeze dried fascia lata allografts. Preliminary studies in a goat model. *Am J Sports Med*, 15, pp. 295–303

Jozsa, L.; Kvist, M. & Balint, B. et al. (1989). The role of recreational sport activity in Achilles tendon rupture: a clinical, pathoanatomical, and sociological study of 292 cases. *Am J Sports Med*, 17, pp. 338-343

Kissel, C.; Blacklidge, D. & Crowley, D. (1994). Repair of neglected Achilles tendon ruptures--procedure and functional results. *J Foot Ankle Surg*, 33, 1, pp. 46-52

Lee, D. (2007). Achilles tendon repair with acellular tissue graft augmentation in neglected ruptures. *J Foot Ankle Surg*, 46, 6, pp. 451-455

Lepow, G. & Green, J. (2006). Reconstruction of a neglected Achilles tendon rupture with an Achilles tendon allograft: a case report, *J Foot Ankle Surg*, 45, 5, pp. 351-355

Leppilahti, J. & Orava, S. (1998). Total Achilles tendon rupture. A review. *Sports Med*, 25, 2, pp. 79-100
Lieberman, J.; Lozman, J.; Czajka, J. & Dougherty, J. (1988). Repair of Achilles tendon rupture with Dacron vascular graft. *Clin Orthop*, 243, pp. 204-208
Lindholm, A. (1959). A new method of operation in subcutaenous ruptureof the Achilles tendon. *Acta Chir Scand,* 117, pp. 261-270
longus tendon transfer/augmentation. *Foot Ankle Int,* 21, 12, pp. 1004-1010
Maffulli, N. & Leadbetter, W. (2005). Free gracilis tendon graft in neglected tears of the Achilles tendon. *Clin J Sport Med*, 15, 2, pp. 56-61
Maffulli, N. (1996). Clinical tests in sports medicine: more on Achilles tendon. *Br J Sports Med,* 30, pp. 250
Maffulli, N.; Waterston, S. & Squair, J. et al. (1999). Changing incidence of Achilles tendon rupture in Scotland: a 15-year study. *Clin J Sport Med,* 9, pp. 157-160
Mahirogullari, M.; Ferguson, C.; Whitlock, P.; Stabile, K. & Poehling, G. (2007). Freeze-dried allografts for anterior cruciate ligament reconstruction. 26, pp. 625-637
Mandelbaum, B.; Myerson, M. & Forster, R. (1995). Achilles tendon ruptures. A new method of repair, early range of motion, and functional rehabilitation. *Am J Sports Med,* 2, pp. 392–395
Mann, R.; Holmes, G. & Seale, K. (1991). Chronic rupture of the Achilles tendon: a new technique of repair. *J Bone Joint Surg,* 73A, pp. 214–219
Martin, R.; Manning, C.; Carcia, C. & Conti, S. (2005). An outcome study of chronic Achilles tendinosis after excision of the Achilles tendon and flexor hallucis longus tendon transfer. *Foot Ankle Int,* 26, 9, pp. 691-697
Mendicino, S. & Reed, T. (1996). Repair of neglected Achilles tendon ruptures with a triceps surae muscle tendon advancement. *J Foot Ankle Surg*, 35, 1, pp. 13-18
Miskulin, M.; Miskulin, A.; Klobucar, H. & Kuvalja, S. (2005). Neglected rupture of the Achilles tendon treated with peroneus brevis transfer: a functional assessment of 5 cases. *J Foot Ankle Surg*, 44, 1, pp. 49-56
Monroe, M.; Dixon, D. & Beals, T. et al. (2000). Plantarfelxion torque following reconstruction of Achilles tendinosis or rupture with flexor hallucis longus augmentation. *Foot Ankle Int*, 21, pp. 324-329
Myerson, M. (2010): Disorders of the Achilles tendon, In: *Reconstruction foot and ankle surgery: management of complications, Second Edition*, pp. 341, Saunders, Philadelphia
Nellas, Z.; Lorder, B. & Wertheimer, S. (1996). Reconstruction of an Achilles tendon defect utilizing an Achilles tendon allograft. *J Foot Ankle Surg,* 35, pp. 144-148
Nillius, S.; Nilsson, B. & Westlin, N (1976). The incidence of Achilles tendon rupture. *Acta Orthop Scand,* 47, 1, pp. 118-121
of chronic Achilles tendinopathy. *Foot Ankle Int,* 24, 9, pp. 673-676
Ozaki, J.; Fujiki, J. & Sugimoto, K. et al. (1989). Reconstruction of the neglected Achilles tendon rupture with Marlex mesh. *Clin Orthop Relat Res*, 238, pp. 204-208
Parsons, J.; Weiss, A. & Schenk, RS. et al. (1989). Long-term follow-up of Achilles tendon repair with an absorbable polymer carbon fiber composite. *Foot Ankle*, 9, 4, pp. 179-184
Pintore, E.; Barra, V.; Pintore, R. & Maffulli, N. (2001). Peroneus brevis tendon transfer in neglected tears of the Achilles tendon. *J Trauma*, 50, 1, pp. 71-78
Platt, H. (1931). Observations on Some Tendon Ruptures. *British Med J*, 1, pp. 611-615

Poehling, G.; Curl, W.; Lee, C.; Ginn, T.; Rushing, J.; Naughton, M.; Holden, M.; Martin, D. & Smith, B. (2005). Analysis of outcomes of anterior cruciate ligament repair with 5 year follow-up: allograft versus autograft. *Arthroscopy,* 21, 7, pp. 774-785

Porter, D.; Mannarino, F.; Snead, D.; Gabel, S. & Ostrowski, M. (1997). Primary repair without augmentation for early neglected Achilles tendon ruptures in the recreational athlete. *Foot Ankle Int,* 18, 9, pp. 557-564

Schedl, R. & Fasol, P. (1979). Achilles tendon repair with the plantaris tendon compared with repair using polyglycol threads. *J Trauma,* 19, pp. 189-194

Schuberth, J.; Dockery, G. & McBride R. (1984). Recurrent rupture of the tendo Achillis: repair by free tendinous autograft. *J Am Podiatr Med Assoc,* 74, pp.157-162

Schuberth, JM, B. (1996):Achilles tendon trauma, In: *Foot and ankle trauma,* Scurran, B. pp. 225, Churchill Livingston, Inc., New York

Shino, K.; Inoue, M.; Horibe, S.; Nagano, J. & Ono, K. (1998). Maturation of allograft tendons transplanted into the knee: an arthroscopic and histological study. *J Bone Joint Surg Br,* 70, pp. 556 -560

Tashjian, R.; Hur, J.; Sullivan, R.; Campbell, J. & DiGiovanni, C. (2003). Flexor hallucis longus transfer for repair

Teuffer, A. (1974). Traumatic rupture of the Achilles tendon: reconstruction by transplant and graft using lateral peroneus brevis. *Orthop Clin North Am,* 5, pp. 89 -93

Turco, V. & Spinella, A. (1987). Achilles tendon ruptures: peroneus brevis transfer. *Foot Ankle,* 7, pp. 253–259

Wapner, K.; Hecht, P. & Mills, R. Jr. (1995). Reconstruction of neglected Achilles tendon injury. *Orthop Clin North Am,* 26, 2, pp. 249-263

Wapner, K.; Pavlock, G. & Hecht, P. et al. (1993). Repair of chronic Achilles tendon rupture with flexor hallucis longus tendon transfer. *Foot Ankle,* 14, 8, pp. 443-449

White, R. & Kraynick, B. (1959). Surgical uses of the peroneus brevis tendon. *Surg Gynecol Obstet,* 108, 1, pp. 117-121

Wilcox, D.; Bohay, D. & Anderson, J. (2000). Treatment of chronic Achilles tendon disorders with flexor hallucis

Yuen, J. & Nicholas, R. (2000). Reconstruction of a total Achilles tendon and soft-tissue defect utilizing an Achilles allograft combined with a rectus muscle free flap. *J Plast Reconstr Surg,* 107, pp. 1807-1811